Fever in Pregnancy

... too hot to handle

Handbook for Obstetricians

Fever in Pregnancy

... too hot to handle

Handbook for Obstetricians

Reena Wani

MD, MRCOG, DNBE, FCPS, DGO, DFP, FICOG

Chairperson
FOGSI Perinatology Committee 2015-2017

Additional Professor and Unit Head
Department of Obstetrics and Gynecology
Hindu Hridaysamrat Balasaheb Thakre Medical College
and Dr RN Cooper Municipal Hospital, Juhu, Mumbai
ex-TN Medical College and BYL Nair Ch Hospital
Mumbai

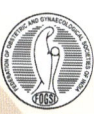 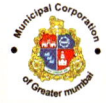

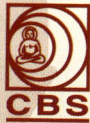

CBS Publishers & Distributors Pvt Ltd

New Delhi • Bengaluru • Chennai • Kochi • Kolkata • Mumbai
Hyderabad • Nagpur • Patna • Pune • Vijayawada

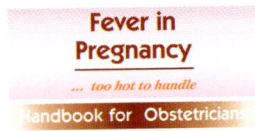

ISBN: 978-81-239-2899-9

First Edition: 2016

Published by Satish Kumar Jain and produced by Varun Jain for
CBS Publishers & Distributors Pvt Ltd
4819/XI Prahlad Street, 24 Ansari Road, Daryaganj, New Delhi 110 002, India.
Ph: 23289259, 23266861, 23266867   Fax: 011-23243014   Website: www.cbspd.com
e-mail: delhi@cbspd.com; cbspubs@airtelmail.in.

Corporate Office: 204 FIE, Industrial Area, Patparganj, Delhi 110 092
Ph: 4934 4934   Fax: 4934 4935   e-mail: publishing@cbspd.com; publicity@cbspd.com

Branches

- **Bengaluru:** Seema House 2975, 17th Cross, K.R. Road, Banasankari 2nd Stage, Bengaluru 560 070, Karnataka
  Ph: +91-80-26771678/79   Fax: +91-80-26771680   e-mail: bangalore@cbspd.com
- **Chennai:** No. 7, Subbaraya Street, Shenoy Nagar, Chennai 600 030, Tamil Nadu
  Ph: +91-44-26680620, 26681266   Fax: +91-44-42032115   e-mail: chennai@cbspd.com
- **Kochi:** Ashana House, 39/1904, AM Thomas Road, Valanjambalam, Ernakulam 682 016, Kochi, Kerala
  Ph: +91-484-4059061–65,67   Fax: +91-484-4059065   e-mail: kochi@cbspd.com
- **Kolkata:** No. 6/B, Ground Floor, Rameswar Shaw Road, Kolkata-700014 (West Bengal), India
  Ph: +91-33-2289-1126, 2289-1127, 2289-1128   e-mail: kolkata@cbspd.com
- **Mumbai:** 83-C, Dr E Moses Road, Worli, Mumbai-400018, Maharashtra
  Ph: +91-22-24902340/41   Fax: +91-22-24902342   e-mail: mumbai@cbspd.com

Representatives

- **Hyderabad** 0-9885175004   • **Nagpur** 0-9021734563   • **Patna**   0-9334159340
- **Pune**   0-9623451994   • **Vijayawada** 0-9000660880

Printed at Magic international Pvt. Ltd., Greater Noida

STILL

The doctor looked worriedly at the reports
and checked the thermometer again,
He wrote something down, looking sad
then put down the pen.

She would never see her child walk, talk or even cry,
Before the child had breathed its first,
It had breathed its last,
and she had to say goodbye ...

They waited with bated breath
For her to wail for the unborn, unseen and unheard
But there was only stunned silence
Not a tear nor a word.

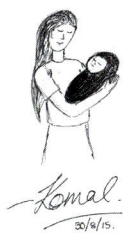

Komal Wani

Foreword

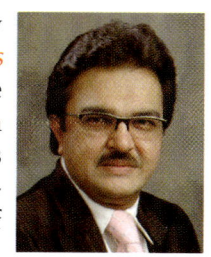

It gives me great pleasure to see this handbook being released in my Presidential year. The theme for this year has been *Minimal Access Maximum Care* and *Pregnancy in High-Risk Mother*. Women with febrile illness in pregnancy fall into this high-risk category. We have focused on high-risk pregnancies in our Hyderabad conference recently which was attended by 2000 delegates. We are also planning to come out with evidence-based guidelines for both obstetric and gynecologic conditions by the end of my Presidential tenure.

As every obstetrician is aiming to have a healthy mother and healthy baby, we need to have a well thought out plan when a problem like fever comes up. I congratulate Dr Reena Wani, Chairperson, Perinatology, who is doing a lot of work in mother and newborn health, for this effort. She has renowned experts in the field to contribute to this handbook which is very practically oriented. I am sure this book will be useful to all FOGSI members.

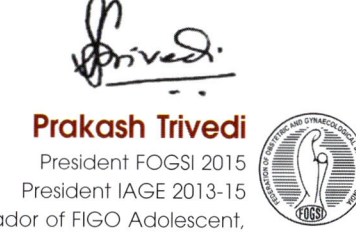

Prakash Trivedi
President FOGSI 2015
President IAGE 2013-15
Regional Ambassador of FIGO Adolescent,
Preconception and Maternal Nutrition Initiative 2015-18

Foreword

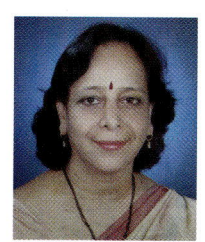

It gives me a great pleasure to see the release of Fever in Pregnancy by Dr Reena Wani who has been working in the Municipal Corporation in the field of Maternal and Child Health since many years.

As Director it is my responsibility and privilege to make many decisions regarding healthcare of women and children amongst other activities to improve health education and awareness. Many specialists working with the BMC have penned down their suggestions and protocols for managing cases with fever due to different causes in pregnant women. This is a vulnerable population and needs special care for good outcome of 2 patients, mother and baby. I have always focused on ways to reduce maternal mortality in the corporation hospitals and febrile illnesses are the important causes which can lead to fatal outcomes if not handled in a timely and appropriate manner.

We need to have an evidence-based approach to treatment but also focus on primary prevention by healthcare measures (sanitation, vector control, infection prevention) and early detection. MCGM has a state-of-the-art laboratory facility in Kasturba Hospital and we hope to develop this infectious disease center further.

I would urge all of you doing work in MCH care to join hands to give optimal and standardized care to our women to make our city and state, the leader in healthcare statistics.

Suhasini Nagda
Director (ME and MH), MCGM, Mumbai
Dean, Nair Hospital Dental College
Immediate Past President, Indian Prosthodontics Society
FDS RCPS, Glasgow
FAIMER FELLOW 2012

Foreword

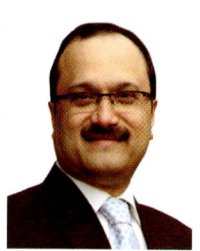

Pregnancy and delivery are the two most stressful events in a woman's life. As obstetricians and caregivers, we take the ultimate responsibility to try and ensure a safe journey to both the mother and the child.

Fever in pregnancy can be very difficult to diagnose and still more difficult to treat, keeping in mind the limitations as far as the diagnostic tools and the treatment modalities are concerned.

I am delighted that now with this book Fever in Pregnancy we will be better equipped to face the situation. Newer diseases are discovered and still newer drugs to combat them are flooding the market, making it very difficult to choose. Hence it is of utmost importance that obstetricians are updated on this situation. This book is an excellent collection of all the various illnesses presenting with fever in pregnancy. Its contents will be of interest even to those outside the specialty, including the internist and infectious disease specialist.

Whether you are a medical student or a postgraduate resident, or even a teaching faculty, you will find this handbook very simple to comprehend with vital information within the covers of this book. I am sure you will enjoy this book as much as I did.

Ameet Patki
MD, DNB, FCPS, FICOG, FRCOG (UK)

Hon Associate Professor
KJ Somaiya Medical College and Hospital
Mumbai

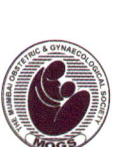

Medical Director
Fertility Associates, Mumbai

Consultant Obstetrician and Gynaecologist
Khar Hinduja Surgicals, Mumbai.

Past President
The Mumbai Obstetric and Gynaecological Society (2014-15)

Preface

Maternal fever is a considerable common problem. This is primarily a cause for concern as we need to deal with two patients—mother and fetus. Depending on the trimester in which the patient presents, our concerns may be different. We may be having the help of physicians and other specialists but as obstetricians we are finally responsible for the patients hence our approach should be systematic and evidence based.

The genesis of this book was at the Annual MOGS Conference in January 2015 when Dr Ameet Patki asked me to conduct a panel discussion on "Fever in Pregnancy"—there was much discussion, debate and interest generated and many requests for written information. That is when the concept of getting the experts to pen down their suggestions was born…and literally 9 months later we are holding the baby in our hands!!

The evaluation and management of febrile illness in pregnancy is sometimes complicated. The reasons include difficulty in interpreting symptoms, concerns about performing imaging and about the complications of therapy in both the mother and the fetus. Decision making is the most important activity in patient management. Over years of training and practice, doctors acquire lots of knowledge and skills. The skills of clinical judgment and its application to individual patient are what distinguish good clinicians from others. We have experts covering this and specific aspects of febrile illnesses in this handbook.

Pregnancy induces a unique challenge for the maternal immune system and invading pathogens can take advantage of these alterations putting women at a higher risk of developing complications. For example in influenza, most patients make a full recovery after a mild flu. However, pregnant women need to be actively treated from the start as they are likely to develop pulmonary complications and swine flu is a notifiable disease.

Pregnancy may change the symptomatology, and extent of affection of the body. For example, hepatitis E is relatively benign in nonpregnant women but associated with high maternal mortality in pregnancy. In pregnancy malaria *P. falciparum* causes greater morbidity and mortality than non-falciparum infections but there is mounting evidence that *P. vivax* is not as benign as had been previously thought. All this is covered in this handbook.

Although maternal fever has been implicated as a human teratogen in several studies, we need to know not only the impact of fever but also the specific affectation due to a particular agent to counsel, treat and manage the case. The infections commonly seen in pregnancy during monsoon have also been covered in detail, along with specific types of diseases.

Theodore Billroth has said:

"It is a most gratifying sign of the rapid progress of our time that our best textbooks become antiquated so quickly."

Hence there is the need to keep updating ourselves with the changes in medical knowledge.

Early medical advice, up-to-date and timely treatment of various febrile illnesses can prevent morbidity and mortality in pregnancy. This handbook has been compiled with inputs from experts in various fields and we are sure it will be helpful to you, dear readers!

Reena Wani

Acknowledgments

I would like to thank the following persons without whom this book would not have been possible.

- My patients over the years at Nair, Kasturba and Cooper Hospitals—each case taught me new things!
- My family especially Varun (budding medical student) and my daughter Komal (budding artist) for condoning the time spent away from them.
- Dean Sir (Dr) RM Chaturvedi for his guidance and support in many ways.
- Ramesh Krishnamachari and Dr Madhuri Mehendale for their constant help and follow-up.
- All the experienced contributors for timely submission of their chapters.

Reena Wani

List of Contributors

Aditya Gupta
Resident, Department of Medicine
Seth GS Medical College & KEM
Hospital
Parel, Mumbai

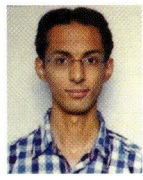

Anahita Chauhan MD, DGO, DFP
Additional Professor and Unit Head
Department of Obstetrics and
Gynecology
Seth GS Medical College & KEM
Hospital, Mumbai
Honorary Consultant, Saifee Hospital
Joint Clinical Secretary, Mumbai Obstetric and
Gynecological Society

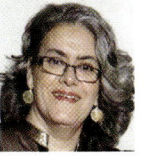

Ankesh R Sahetya DGO, DNB
Speciality Medical Consultant
Bandra Bhabha Hospital
Mumbai, Maharashtra

Arun Nayak
Professor and Head of Unit
Department of Obstetrics and
Gynecology
Lokmanya Tilak Medical College
and General Hospital, Sion
President, Mumbai Obstetrics
and Gynecology Society
Secretary and Manager, The Journal of
Obstetrics and Gynecology of India

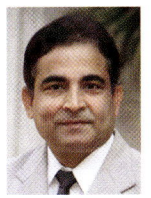

Avinash Supe MS, FICS, DNBE, FCPS,
DHA, PGDME, MHPE (UIC) FIAGES, FMAS,
FAIS
Dean, GS Medical College KEM
Hospital
Professor, GI Surgery
Director, GSMC FAIMER regional
Institute
Immediate Past President, IHPBA-India
Ex Dean–Sion Hospital

Chitra Nayak
Professor and Head, Department
of Dermatology
BYL Nair Charitable Hospital and
TN Medical College, Mumbai

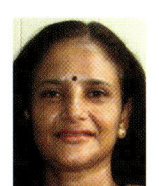

Dhananjay Ogale MD
Assistant Professor, Department of
Medicine
HBTMC and Dr RN Cooper Hospital,
Mumbai Maharashtra

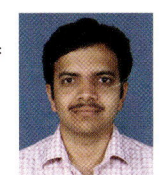

Divya Sahetya MS
Consultant Obstetrician and
Gynecologist
Pushpaa Hospital

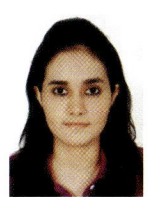

Jayanthi Shastri
Professor and Head
Department of Microbiology
TN Medical College and BYL Nair
Charitable Hospital, Mumbai,
Maharashtra

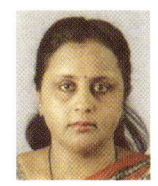

Kartikeya Bhagat MD, FICOG, IBCLC
Consultant Obstetrician and
Gynecologist
Grace Maternity and Nursing
Home, Kandivli West, Mumbai
Past President, Association of
Fellow Gynecologists (AFG)
International Board Certified Lactation
Consultant (IBCLC)

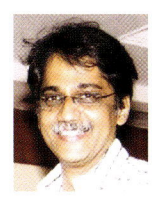

Khushboo Bagdi MS DNB
Consultant Obstetrician and
Gynecologist
Mumbai, Maharashtra

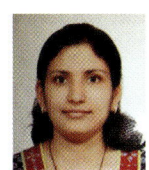

Madhva Prasad MS
Senior Registrar LTMG and Hospital
Sion, Mumbai

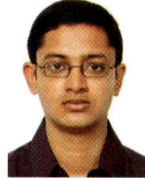

Madhuri Mehendale
Assistant Professor
Lokmanya Tilak Medical College
and General Hospital, Sion
Managing Council Member
Mumbai Obstetrics and
Gynecology Society

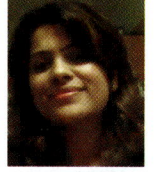

Maitri C Shah
Associate Professor
Dept. of Obstetrics and Gynecology
Medical College and SSG Hospital
Baroda

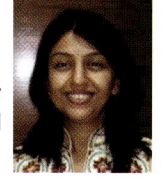

Namrata Mehta MS, DGO, DNB
Assistant Professor, Department of
Obstetrics and Gynecology
NowrosjeeWadia Hospital, Parel
Mumbai, Maharashtra

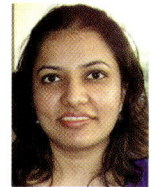

Neelam N Redkar MD
Professor, Dept of Medicine
HBTMC and Dr RN Cooper
Hospital, Juhu Mumbai

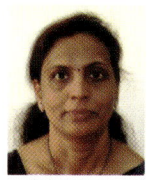

Niteen D Karnik
Professor and I/C MICU
Department of Medicine
Seth GS Medical College and KEM
Hospital, Parel, Mumbai 400012

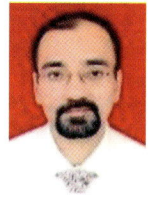

Om Shrivastav
Director, Infectious Diseases Clinic
Jaslok Hospital and Research
Centre,15, Deshmukh Marg
Pedder Road, Mumbai

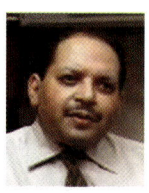

Parikshit D Tank MD DNB FCPS DGO
DFP MNAMS MICOG MRCOG
Chairperson, Safe Motherhood
Committee, FOGSI
Nowrosjee Wadia Maternity
Hospital
Ashwini Maternity and Surgical
Hospital
Center for Endoscopy and Assisted Reproduction
Jupiter Hospital

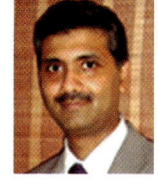

Pradnya Supe MS
Assistant Professor
Department of Obstetrics and
Gynecology
Lokmanya Tilak Municipal
Medical College, Sion, Mumbai
Maharashtra

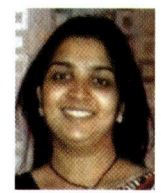

Prakash Ram Relwani, MD
Assistant Professor
Dept of Medicine
HBTMC and Dr RN Cooper
Hospital, Juhu Mumbai

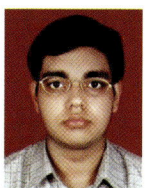

Preeta R Yadav MD, DDV, DNB, FAAD
Dermatologist and Cosmetologist
Director
Skin Health Clinic, Shivaji Park
Mumbai
Consultant, SL Raheja Fortis
Hospital, Mahim, Mumbai
Maharashtra

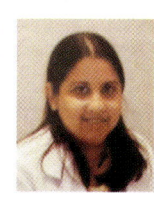

Preeti Yogesh Bhandari MS, DNB,
MICOG, DRM (Germany), PGDMLS
Specialist Gynecologist
Corniche Hospital, Abu Dhabi
UAE Ex Assistant Professor TN
Medical College, Mumbai
Ex Consultant Fertility Specialist
Rotunda IVF Center, Mumbai

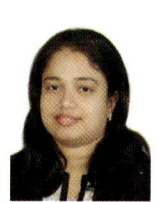

Rachna Bhagat MD, DGO, IBCLC
Consultant Obstetrician and
Gynecologist, Grace Maternity
and Nursing Home, Kandivli West
Mumbai Maharashtra
International Board Certified
Lactation Consultant (IBCLC)

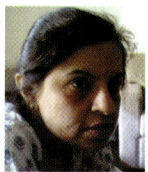

Rashmi Jalvee MS, DGO, DNB
Assistant Professor Department of Obstetrics and Gynecology HBTMC and Dr RN Cooper Hospital Mumbai, Maharashtra

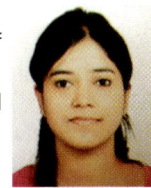

Sarita Agrawal
Professor and Head, Department of Obstetrics and Gynecology, All India Institute of Medical Sciences Raipur (CG)

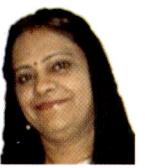

Reena Wani (MD, MRCOG, DNBE, FCPS, DGO, DFP, FICOG)
Chairperson FOGSI Perinatology Committee 2015–2017
Professor Addl and Unit Head, Dept of Obstetrics and Gynecology HBTMC and Dr RN Cooper Hospital, Mumbai, Maharashtra Ex-TN Medical College and BYL Nair Ch Hospital, Mumbai

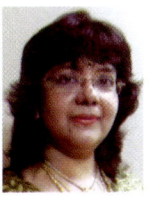

Saurabh Dani
West Zone Co-ordinator, FOGSI Perinatology Committee
Jt. Secretary, ISPAT Treasure Association of Fellow Gynecologists
Co-Founder, Health N Wellness Co-Founder and Director, Prenatal Care and Support LLP

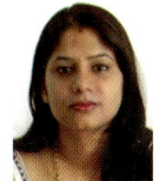

Ramesh M Chaturvedi MD
Dean, HBTMC and Dr. RN Cooper Hospital, Mumbai, Maharashtra

Shreya Goenka
Senior Resident, Department of Obstetrics and Gynecology, All India Institute of Medical Sciences, Raipur (CG)

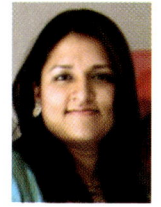

Saloni Prajapati
Assistant Professor
Dept of Obstetrics and Gynecology GMERS Medical College and Gotri Hospital Baroda

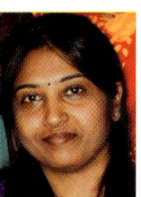

Shreya Prabhoo MBBS, DGO, DNB
Assistant Professor, Dept of Obstetrics and Gynecology Topiwala National Medical College, and BYL Nair Hospital

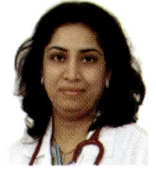

Sandhya Sawant
Assistant Professor, Department of Microbiology
TN Medical College and BYL Nair Charitable Hospital, Mumbai Maharashtra

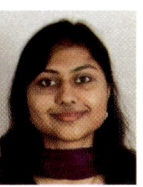

Shruti Bangale Daflapurkar
Specialist Obstetrician and Gynecologist
Orion Family Medical Centre, Dubai

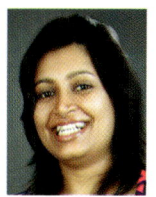

Sanjay W Gulhane
Associate Professor, Department of Medicine
HBTMC and Dr RN Cooper Hospital, Juhu, Mumbai, Maharashtra

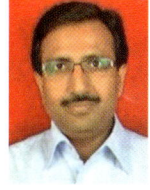

Shruti Thar
DGO Resident, Department of Obstetrics and Gynecology Nowrosjee Wadia Hospital, Parel Mumbai, Maharashtra

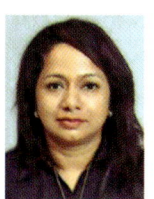

Sanjay B Prabhu MD DCH IBCLC
Director, Neoplus Criticare Children Hospital
Borivali, Mumbai

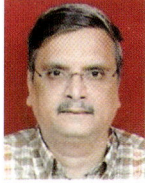

Sophia D Fernandes MD, DPH
Assistant Professor, Department of Community Medicine, HBTMC Dr RN Cooper Hospital, Juhu, Mumbai Maharashtra

Unnati Desai
Assistant Professor
Department of Pulmonary
Medicine
TN Medical College and BYL Nair
Hospital
Mumbai, Maharashtra

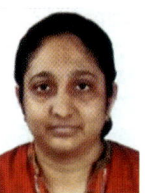

Vinaya S Karkhanis
Additional Professor
Department of Pulmonary
Medicine
TN Medical College and
BYL Nair Hospital
Mumbai, Maharashtra

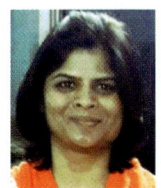

Contents

Section III Specific Situations

Section IV Specific Diseases in Pregnancy

Section

I

Overview

Art and Science of Clinical Decision Making in Gynecology and Obstetrics

Pradnya Supe, Avinash Supe

Decision making is the most important activity in patient management. Over years of training and practice, doctors acquire lots of knowledge and skills. The skills of clinical judgment and its application to individual patient are what distinguish good clinician from others. During last few years this has become more relevant as patients are increasingly becoming partners in a shared decision-making process. Clinical decision making is defined as systematic, explicative and quantitative way of making decisions in healthcare. When one considers science of "decision making", there are many issues and beliefs that one has to understand or assume.

Though every specialty in medicine is different, large majority of clinical decisions are variations of basic patterns of decision making problems that are similar across specialties and amenable to the same basic classes of conceptual tools. All carpenters apply a common set of tools to a common raw material. A master carpenter, however, produces valuable and unique piece by critically evaluating the distinctive grain of a piece of wood carefully, choosing which tools are appropriate, and skilfully applying those tools to the best effect. A master clinician similarly achieves great results for patients by considering each patient as a unique individual and selectively applying conceptual tool in a skilful manner.

Secondly, it is important to understand that making good decisions is more important in practice than making perfect decisions. Science can offer many treatments and journals may quote excellent results but a good clinician will always select what suits to his/her patients considering cost, culture and usefulness (best available rather than best possible). Thirdly many clinical decisions require input from both physicians and patients, but physicians and patients are not inter-changeable. Each brings a unique perspective and unique information that is largely inaccessible to the other—a point that is often made when physicians write about their experiences as patients. It is important to consider how much and what kind of information must be provided by the patient in different types of decisions to make the decision process successful. Lastly one has to remember that the practice of medicine and healthcare policy are inseparably linked. Acts of clinical care are influenced by public policy and social context; in many important cases, acts of clinical care may even be expressions of policy. When healthcare demand exceeds resources, when access to care is difficult or inequitable, or when other factors conspire to constrain physician's abilities to provide excellent care, they often become advocates not only for their individual patients, but also for the health of their society. Any healthcare decision affects an individual patient as well as that has impact on the patients, family, community, and society. There is need for scientific approach to medical decision making in our country.

Medical or clinical decision making is a new specialty established in developed world. One wonders how clinicians take decisions. In routine clinical practice majority (80–85%) of our decisions are based on hypothesis. After a thorough clinical examination and history, we think of differential diagnosis based on combinations of various symptoms and signs and its occurrence in particular disease. With process of heuristic decision making (hypo-thesis), we make a tentative diagnosis that is confirmed with investigations. Other decision-making processes include algorithmic (15–20%) and intuitive decision making (less than 5%). This is not technical rationality but also close attention to the values and goals of thoughtful clinical practice.

PROACTIVE approach to decision making:
- Problem—define the problem
- Reframe—reframe from multiple pers-pectives
- Objective—focus on the objective
- Alternatives—consider all relevant alternative treatments
- Consequences and chances
- Trade-offs—identify and estimate value trade offs
- Integrate—integrate the evidence and values
- Value—optimize

INTERPRETING DIAGNOSTIC TESTS

In daily practice we do not develop new diagnostic tests. Instead we select from available tests with recommended thresholds. The selection is based ideally, on the characteristics of the test (sensitivity and specificity) and the decision that will be taken depending on the test result. Patients are rarely interested in the sensitivity of the test—what proportion of sick people test positive.

Their main concern is the meaning of a positive (or a negative) test to them is of those who test positive, what proportion is actually sick? The latter is also expressed as the "predicted probability of a positive test" or positive predictive value; and it depends not only on the sensitivity and specificity of the test, but also on the prior (before-testing) likelihood that the patient was sick. When a condition is rare, or the patient is unlikely to have the condition because of other clinical factors, the positive predictive value of a test for the condition will be lower than if the condition is common or the patient has other factors that increase suspicion of the condition.

MULTIPLE TESTS

In some cases, a single diagnostic test may not be sufficient to warrant action. For example, if the treatment is invasive, and the test is imperfect, may not be comfortable treating patients because the false positive rate is high. In this situation, it is common to combine the results of multiple tests. Often the tests are chosen so that one has high sensitivity and the other has high specificity; together, the test results serve to effectively diagnose the condition.

COMBINING RESULTS

A good example of combining tests is blood testing for HIV infection. HIV testing typically includes a highly sensitive ELISA screening test paired with a highly specific Western blot test or two different methods of ELISA.

STRATEGIES FOR ORDERING TESTS IN GYNECOLOGY

Decision analysis has frequently been applied to compare alternative diagnostic workup strategies. For example, Gracia and Barnhart (2001)[1] compared six strategies for diagnosing ectopic pregnancy in women presenting with abdominal pain or bleeding in their first trimester:

1. Ultrasound followed by serum quantitative hCG
2. hCG followed by ultrasound
3. Serum progesterone followed by ultrasound followed by hCG
4. Progesterone followed by hCG followed by ultrasound
5. Ultrasound followed by repeat ultrasound
6. Clinical examination alone

Assuming that the primary goal was not to miss an ectopic pregnancy (that is, to have a low rate of false negatives), the study found that the first two strategies and the repeat ultrasound would maximize the sensitivity of the workup, detecting 100% of ectopic pregnancies. However, because the initial ultrasound is slightly better at ruling out ectopic pregnancy on its own than other initial tests, strategy 1 (ultrasound followed by serum hCG) would result in fewer false positives (leading to interrupted intrauterine pregnancies, some of which may have been viable) than the other two; its specificity was about 99%, whereas the others were about 98%.

Diagnosis is rightly considered one of the most important aspects of clinical decision making. Diagnostic tests are developed to fit particular decisions; the choice of the test depends in large part on the goals of the clinician. Clinicians have a variety of measures by which the performance of a test may be assessed, and formal tools exist to use test results to help clinicians support their beliefs in patients assumed diagnosis. In the absence of formal methods, a powerful system of intuition guides judgement and can be both improved and checked by formal reasoning.

QUALITY ADJUSTED LIFE EXPECTANCY

For each year (or month, or day) of the patients life, add up the quality associated with the state of health he/she will experience that year, discounted by her health discount rate say 3% annually if the state will be experienced in the future. The resulting number is the patient's quality adjusted life expectancy.[2]

The difference in QALY between any two treatment options is a measure of benefit of one treatment over the other.

Usefulness and Limitations of QALY

Measuring the effects of treatments in terms of QALY is very useful, because QALY's provide a single measure of effectiveness that can be compared across a variety of treatments for diverse health problems. This is particularly useful when making decisions that offer trade-offs between length and quality of life. Every clinician and patient must understand these trade-offs while adopting newer therapies and drugs in clinical practice.

Although QALY'S provide a useful model for the impact of treatments on patients' lives, they necessarily involve simplification of how a health profile will be experienced. QALY's do not incorporate any information (beyond simple discounting) about the sequence of health states that will occur. They also present challenges when used to make policy decisions.

UNCERTAINTY IN DECISION MAKING

It reflects our inability to know anything with complete surety. This inability is associated with anxiety, doubt and perhaps lack of knowledge. It is also the engine of excitability and may lead to new discoveries.

The most common uncertainty encountered in medical practice is "risk". "Risk" refers to uncertainty about the state of the world that can be precisely quantified as probability. This is the form of uncertainty that the gamblers experience while playing roulette. When considering patient behaviour, subjective risk—the risk as perceived by patient is often more important than objective risk the best estimate of risk from epidemiological and pathophysiological data.

Another common type of uncertainty present in many medical decisions occurs when the state of the world is unknown and cannot be precisely quantified as a probability. Instead one may be able to provide only a range of probabilities or a more qualitative statement that the event is likely or unlikely. This type of uncertainty is also called ambiguity.

One more uncertainty is when there is personal lack of knowledge. When a physician considers problems outside his or her area of expertise or familiar territory; he or she may have a vague idea of treatments, outcomes but without further study or consultation; he or she will be unable to provide precise estimate of probabilities.

RATIONAL AND ETHICAL DECISION MAKING IN OBSTETRICS AND GYNECOLOGY[3]

Ethical Principles

The major principles that act as guides to professional action and for resolving conflicting obligations in healthcare are respect for autonomy, beneficence and non-maleficence and justice. Other principles are fidelity, honesty, privacy and confidentiality.

a. *Respect for autonomy:* It literally means self-rule. It implies personal rule of self that is free both from controlling interferences by others and from personal limitations that prevent meaningful choice. It acknowledges an individual's right to hold views, to make choices and to take actions based on her own personal beliefs.

b. *Beneficence and non-maleficence:* Beneficence literally means doing or producing good, expresses the obligation to promote the well-being of others. It requires a physician to act in a way that is likely to benefit the patient. Non-maleficence is the obligation to not to harm or cause injury. They are both considered manifestations of the same principle.

c. *Justice:* Principle of rendering to others what is due to them. It deals with not only the physician's obligation to render to a patient what is owed but also with the physicians role in the allocation of limited medical resources in the broader community.

Obstetrician–gynecologists, like other physicians, often face a conflict between principles of beneficence–non-maleficence in relation to a patient and respect for that patient's personal autonomy. In such cases, the physician's judgment about what is in the patient's best interests conflicts with the patient's preferences. The physician then has to decide whether to respect the patient's choices or to refuse to act on the patient's preferences in order to achieve what the physician believes to be a better outcome for the patient. However, the model of following patients' choices, whatever they are, as long as they are informed choices, also has been criticized for reducing the physician to a mere technician.[4] Other models have been proposed, such as negotiation,[5] shared decision making[6], or a deliberative model, in which the physician integrates information about the patient's condition with the patient's values to make a cogent recommendation. Whatever model is selected, a physician may still, in a particular situation, have to decide whether to act on the patient's request that does not appear to accord with the patient's best interests.

THE UNESCO ETHICAL METHOD OF REASONING[7]

First step	Fact deliberation—analyse the case/deliberation about medical facts
Second step	Value deliberation—identify moral problems and conflict of values
Third step	Duty deliberation—identify course of action/reflecting on the most challenging cases/reflecting on other cases
Fourth step	Testing consistency—guard against inconsistency by using the law and opinion of other experts
Fifth step	Conclusion—arrive at wise decisions

CASE SCENARIO

A 26-year-old Primi Para requests to be delivered by cesarean section because she does not want to undergo the pain associated with normal labour. She is averagely built and is healthy otherwise. This pregnancy is uncomplicated. There are no obstetrical indications for cesarean section.

Reasoning and Ethical Decision-making[8]

Fact deliberation: The term cesarean delivery on maternal request (CDMR) refers to elective delivery by cesarean section (CS) at the request of a woman with no identifiable maternal or fetal indications.[9] Major and minor morbidity associated with elective CS has been reviewed systematically in the recent National Institute of Health and Clinical Excellence (NICE) guidelines 2012[10]on Cesarean section, which concluded that there is very little quality evidence to suggest that risks from elective CS are lower or higher than that of a planned vaginal delivery.

Value deliberation: The patient is exercising her autonomy in deciding how she wishes to deliver her child. Maternal autonomy as a central tenet of obstetrical decision making has been reinforced in both law and ethics. However, the doctor has a professional duty to ensure no or minimal harm befalls their patient in the course of treatment. There are concerns that the planned cesarean delivery requested by the patient may pose more harm to her than a planned vaginal delivery in view of a long list of potential morbidities related to the surgery. In public funded healthcare systems, doctor has an ethical duty to community to allocate healthcare resources wisely to procedures and treatment for which there is clear evidence of a net benefit to health.

Duty deliberation: Risks and benefits of the requested procedure should be discussed with the patient and assessment should be made to ascertain that patient is able to demonstrate an understanding of the same. Availability of health resources should also be considered in resource-limited areas. Healthcare provider should offer prenatal childbirth education, emotional support in labour and anesthesia for child birth if fear of pain during child birth persists.[9]

Testing consistency: At present there is no hard evidence on the relative risks and benefits of term cesarean delivery for non-medical reasons, as compared with vaginal delivery, i.e. no evidence from randomised controlled trials upon which to base any practice recommendations regarding CDMR.[11] However, available evidence suggests that normal vaginal delivery is safer in the short and long term for both mother and child. Surgery on the uterus also has implications for later pregnancies and deliveries. At present, because hard evidence of net benefit does not exist, performing CS for non-medical reasons is ethically not justified.[12] However, while performing CS for non-medical reasons a decade ago was considered ethically not justified, recent guidelines seem much more supportive of women's choices.[13] The NICE guidelines on CS recognises that a better approach than counselling women requesting CS about the risks would be to explore, record and discuss the reasons for the request, thereby individualising cases and management.[10]

Conclusion/decision: Cesarean section upon maternal requests can be performed if the patient is able to demonstrate sufficient understanding of risks and benefits of the procedure, including the long term risks, and the physician believes there are no significant health concerns for the mother and fetus and cost factor does not play a major role. ACOG committee recommends that in case of cesarean section on maternal request; it should not be performed before 39 weeks of gestational age; should not be motivated by unavailability of pain management; and should not be recommended for women desiring multiple children, given that risks of placenta previa, accreta and gravid hysterectomy increase with each cesarean delivery.[9]

SUMMARY

Clinical decision making is both art and science. Understanding science of clinical decision making facilitates an artful clinician to make rational and ethical decisions. This is more so with gynecologist and obstetricians who deals with more complex problems with social and cultural backgrounds. Obstetrician–gynecologists who are familiar with the concepts of medical ethics will be better able to approach complex ethical situations in a clear and structured way. By considering the ethical frameworks involving principles, virtues, care and feminist perspectives, concern for community, and case precedents, they can enhance their ability to make ethically justifiable clinical decisions.

REFERENCES

1. Gracia CR,Barnhart KT. Diagnosing ectopic pregnancy: Decision analysis comparing six strategies Obstet Gynecol 2001 Mar; 97(3):464–70.
2. Schwartz Alan and Bergus George "Quality and Quantity" in Schwartz Alan and Bergus George Eds "Medical Decision Making : A Physicians guide" 2008, Cambridge Press, New York, Pp 43–51.
3. ACOG committee guidelines no 397 Dec 2007 (Reaffirmed 2013) from http://www.acog.org/ Resources-And-Publications/accessed on 27th April 2015.
4. Emanuel EJ, Emanuel LL. Four models of the physician–patient relationship. JAMA 1992;267: 2221–6.
5. Childress JF, Siegler M. Metaphors and models of doctor–patient relationships: Their implications for autonomy. Theor Med 1984;5:17–30.
6. Katz J. The silent world of doctor and patient. Baltimore (MD): Johns Hopkins University Press; 2002.
7. Bioethics core curriculum, UNICEF 2008 from http://unesdoc.unesco.org/ accessed on 29th April 2015.
8. Idris N, Nalliah S . The ethical decision making model in Obstetrics and Gynecology practice International E-Journal of Science, Medicine & Education; 2014, Vol. 8 Issue 1, p44
9. ACOG committee guidelines No. 559 April 2013 from http://www.acog.org/Resources-And-Publications/ accessed on 27th April 2015.
10. NICE guidelines [CG132] on Cesarean section; Published date : November 2011
11. Lavender T, Hofmeyr GJ, Neilson JP, Kingdon C, Gyte GM. Cesarean section for non-medical reasons at term. Cochrane Database Syst Rev. 2006; 3: CD004660.
12. Ethical Issues in Obstetrics and Gynecology by the FIGO Committee for the Study of Ethical Aspects of Human Reproduction and Women's Health. October 2012.
13. Schenker JG, Cain JM. FIGO Committee Report. FIGO Committee for the Ethical Aspects of Human Reproduction and Women's Health. Ethical aspects regarding cesarean delivery for non-medical reasons. Int J Gynaecol Obstet. 1999; 64: 317–22.

2

Epidemiology and Importance of Fever in Pregnant Women

Sophia D Fernandes, RM Chaturvedi

Pregnancy is a dynamic state of health and disease, shared by the pregnant woman and a growing fetus, a concern to the treating physician for timely diagnosis and necessary interventions.[1]

Fever in pregnancy refers to an elevated temperature, often associated with other symptoms, in a woman who is pregnant.

Any acute or chronic infectious diseases may be contracted during the course of pregnancy, and conception may occur in women already subject to infection.

Infections with viral, bacterial, parasitic and fungi do occur in any pregnant woman like other non-pregnant woman of similar age. Most infections are not serious. But some infections are more important in pregnant woman than in non-pregnant woman because of the potential for vertical transmission to foetus or infant.[1]

Also physiological and metabolic changes occurring in pregnancy sometimes precipitate auto-immune complex resulting in non-specific fevers.

CAUSES OF FEVER IN PREGNANCY

Infectious Diseases

1. Tuberculosis in a country like India where TB is an endemic, the pregnant woman is most susceptible to the disease owing to her compromised immune status.
2. Urinary tract infection—Urinary tract infections (UTIs) are common during pregnancy. Increased bladder volume, and decreased bladder tone, along with decreased ureteral tone, contributes to increased urinary stasis and uretero-vesical reflux. Increases in urinary progestins and estrogens may lead to a decreased ability of the lower urinary tract to resist invading bacteria.[8]
3. Respiratory infections (URTI/LRTI)
4. Gastrointestinal infection—appendicitis, diverticulitis, viral diarrhea
5. Vector borne diseases—malaria, dengue, chikungunya
6. Enteric fever
7. Hepatitis
8. Abscesses—hepatic, dental, breast (mastitis)
9. Amebiasis
10. Leptospirosis
11. STI
12. Meningitis

Non-infectious Causes

1. Neoplasms
2. Connective tissue disease—rheumatic fever, rheumatoid arthritis
3. Autoimmune diseases—inflammatory bowel disease, systemic lupus erythematosus
4. Drugs—drugs like beta-lactam antibiotics, procainamide, isoniazid, alpha-methyldopa,

quinidine and diphenylhydantoin are associated with fever. Biological agents like interferons and interleukins used in therapy could also cause fever.

5. Miscellaneous—sarcoidosis, physiological—due to increase in metabolism during pregnancy.

Agent Factors

Viral

a. Enteroviruses
b. Hepatitis E, B, C, D
c. Herpes simplex
d. Human immunodeficiency virus (HIV 1 and 2)
e. Influenza
f. Mumps (myxovirus parotiditis)
g. Measles
h. Rubella (German measles)
i. Varicella zoster (chickenpox)
j. Cytomegalovirus
k. Dengue
l. Chikungunya

Bacterial

a. *Treponema pallidum*
b. *Mycobacterium tuberculosis*
c. *Salmonella typhi/paratyphi*
d. *Staphylococus*
e. *Streptococcus*
f. *Neisseria*

Protozoal

a. *Toxoplasma gondii*
b. *Plasmodium* species

Fungal

Chlamydia trachomatis

Host Factors

One of the most intriguing puzzles in modern immunology involves the "paradox of pregnancy," in which immunologic tolerance to paternally derived fetal antigens is achieved despite an apparently adequate maternal defense against infection. With 50% of its genetic material derived from its father, the fetus's susceptibility to rejection by the maternal immune system is similar to the susceptibility of a transplanted organ. Evidence indicates that the maternal immune system may tolerate fetal antigens by suppressing cell-mediated immunity while retaining normal humoral immunity. These changes are known to occur locally at the maternal-fetal interface but may also affect systemic immune responses to infection. Although pregnant women are not immunosuppressed in the classic sense, immunologic changes of pregnancy may induce a state of increased susceptibility to certain intracellular pathogens, including viruses, intracellular bacteria, and parasites.[2]

Environmental Factors

All factors contributing to transmission of infections need to be considered, i.e. population density and movement, seasonal trends of diseases, weather conditions (rainfall, humidity, temperature), socio-economic conditions, poor housing conditions (overcrowding, poor ventilation), poor sanitation (open air defecation, pollution of drinking water, low standard of food and personal hygiene), high risk behavior, health ignorance.[3]

SYMPTOMS

A body temperature of more than 37.2°C or 98.9°F in the morning or a temperature of more than 37.7° or 99.9°F in the evening indicates fever.

Fever accompanied by any of the following syndromes deserves further scrutiny, because it may indicate an important disease which could leave a long lasting impact on the mother and child:

- (1) Skin rash (2) Difficulty breathing (3) Shortness of breath (4) Persistent cough (5) Decreased consciousness

- (6) Bruising or unusual bleeding (without previous injury) (7) Persistent diarrhea (8) Persistent vomiting (other than air or motion sickness) (9) Jaundice (10) Paralysis of recent onset.

Clinical findings	Infections
Fever and rash	Dengue, chikungunya, rickettsial infections, enteric fever (skin lesions may be sparse or absent), acute HIV infection, measles
Fever, abdominal pain and diarrhea	Enteric fever, amebic liver abscess, inflammatory bowel disease, food poisoning, amoebiasis
Undifferentiated fever and normal or low	Dengue, malaria, rickettsial infection, enteric fever, white blood cell count chikungunya
Fever and hemorrhage	Viral hemorrhagic fevers (dengue and others), meningococcemia, leptospirosis, rickettsial infections
Fever and eosinophilia	Acute schistosomiasis, drug hypersensitivity reaction
Fever and pulmonary infiltrates	Common bacterial and viral pathogens, tuberculosis, leptospirosis, sarcoidosis
Fever and altered mental status	Cerebral malaria, viral or bacterial meningoencephalitis
Fever persisting >2 weeks	Malaria, enteric fever, acute HIV, tuberculosis

EFFECTS

The effects of fever on pregnancy depend on the extent of temperature elevation, its duration, and the stage of fetal development when it occurs. Mild exposures during the preimplantation period and more severe exposures during embryonic and fetal development could result in miscarriage, premature labor, growth restriction, and stillbirth.

High core body temperature, hyperthermia, has been shown in animal models to be a potent teratogen.

Professor Marshall J. Edwards at the University of Sydney, Australia, is generally considered to be the individual who pioneered the discovery that maternal hyperthermia during pregnancy can be teratogenic. His doctoral thesis was entitled "A Study of Some Factors Affecting Fertility of Animals with Particular Reference to the Effects of Hyperthermia on Gestation and Prenatal Development of the Guinea-Pig". In animal studies over the course of 40 years, Edwards demonstrated that mechanisms for hyperthermia-induced fetal damage included cell death, membrane disruption, vascular disruption, and placental infarction. Modest elevations in temperature prior to implantation and more sustained elevations during early embryogenesis may cause fetal death and abortion. Embryos surviving maternal hyperthermia during early development are at risk for a host of congenital anomalies, including neural tube and central nervous system (CNS) defects, microencephaly, microphthalmia, cataracts, craniofacial, heart, renal, dental, and abdominal wall defects among others. The most common cause of hyperthermia during pregnancy is fever related to viral illnesses (and other common causes include bacterial infections associated with pyelonephritis, tonsillitis, and appendicitis).[4]

Following this many animal studies have shown that neural tube and other developmental anomalies occur in the guinea pig following maternal hyperthermia during early neural tube development.[5]

Although animal studies have indicated that fever in pregnancy impacts embryogenesis leading to congenital anomalies and even fetal death, it is extremely difficult if not practically impossible to replicate the same findings on field. In experimental conditions the thermal load variables (temperature change, temperature, time) can be regulated, in real biological conditions these are extremely variable including the additional variables of absolute time of exposure and developmental stage.

A study conducted in the population-based large dataset of the Hungarian Case-Control Surveillance of Congenital Abnormalities, showed an association between high fever-related maternal diseases during the second and/or third gestational months and a higher risk of multiple congenital abnormalities (MCA).[6]

A team of UC Davis researchers has found that mothers who had fevers during their pregnancies were more than twice as likely to have a child with autism or developmental delay than were mothers of typically developing children, and that taking medication to treat fever countered its effect. Published online in the Journal of Autism and Developmental Disorders, the study is believed to be the first to consider how fever from any cause, including the flu, and its treatment during pregnancy could affect the likelihood of having a child with autism or developmental delay.[7]

Hyperthermia in humans (greater than $39.5°C/103°F$) during the first trimester increases the risk of a miscarriage and neural defects.

Although at present it is difficult to explain the exact impact of the fever occurring in pregnancy on the fetus, it is fair enough to say that hyperthermia in pregnancy does have an effect on the fetal development.

In general, perinatal infections have more severe fetal consequences when they occur early in gestation, because first-trimester infections may disrupt organogenesis. Second- and third-trimester infections can cause neurologic impairment or growth disturbances.

CLINICAL EVALUATION AND DIAGNOSIS

In all pregnant women, as in non-pregnant cases, there should be a complete history and physical examination. The examination should be "from head-to-toe"; with special note of the characteristics of the fever, maximum temperature, presence of diurnal variation, and recent travel. The challenge to the clinician is to select investigations with the highest sensitivity and specificity to increase the probability of a correct diagnosis. When the diagnosis continues to be elusive, repeat the history and the physical examination. In cases of a fever in which the cause is unclear, a number of tests may be useful, depending on history and physical examination findings.[8]

PREVENTION AND CONTROL

Primary Prevention

1. Pre-Pregnancy Counselling

Ideally, all women should consult their health-care provider before conception. Pre-pregnancy testing for infections should include an assessment of rubella immunity, syphilis status, human immunodeficiency virus (HIV) status, and immunity to hepatitis B. Some countries test for varicella IgG antibody to exclude previous infection with chickenpox.

Women who lack immunity to rubella, hepatitis B, or varicella, can be advised to have inoculation, and pregnancy should be postponed for at least two months after completion of the vaccination.

2. Antenatal Screening

Screening tests for sexually transmitted infections that are recommended for pregnant women include HIV, hepatitis B, syphilis, and *Chlamydia trachomatis*. Women at risk should be tested for *Neisseria gonorrhea* and hepatitis C.

3. Counselling and Health Education

i. A pre-pregnancy visit is also an opportunity to give dietary and other advice on how to reduce the risk of contracting amoebiasis, hepatitis or food poisoning, i.e. avoid raw or undercooked meat and meat products; peel or wash raw fruit and vegetables thoroughly to remove contaminating soil, and to wash hands after disposing of cat litter or gardening.

ii. The pre-pregnancy session also provides an opportunity for counselling of both partners to avoid casual sexual contact, and intravenous drug use and consequent risk of infection.

iii. *Counselling* during the antenatal period regarding diet, exercise, rest, stress management and avoiding alcohol, smoking and unnecessary drugs.

iv. *Dietary advice*—the diet during pregnancy not only helps in improving the nutritional status of the mother and the foetus but also helps in improving the immunity of the mother. Pregnant women should be advised to avoid raw or undercooked meat, avoid sharing food or drinks with other people. In particular, unpasteurized dairy products, under-cooked meat, and cold meats can contain bacteria that may be harmful for pregnant women. A diet rich in whole foods supports immunity. Fruits and vegetables as fresh garlic, green leafy vegetables, fresh citrus, carotenoids increase the immunity of the mother. Foods rich in essential fatty acids like flax seeds, nuts and seeds should be consumed. Minimize fatty foods such as fast food burgers, as well as sugar and refined flours (breads), caffeinated products and potentially allergic foods such as shellfish. Most importantly pregnant women should strictly consume home cooked food and should avoid eating street food or food cooked outside.

v. *Sexually transmitted infections:* Using of condoms during pregnancy to reduce the risk of STI. Pregnant women should avoid having sex, even with a condom, if the male partner has signs of a sexually transmitted infection.

vi. Pregnant women should take precautions that reduce the risk of acquiring mosquito-borne infections.

vii. *Exercise:* Women who exercise tend to have more appropriate weight gain, less symptomatic pain, decreased gestational diabetes, improved blood pressure control, improvement in immune system response. A regular exercise programme benefits the cardiovascular system, improves blood flow, flushes toxins, keeps endocrine system working well, circulates antibodies, and reduces stress.

viii. Keeping a *positive attitude* and preventing stress are crucial to maintaining a healthy immune system.

Secondary Prevention

Pregnant women should undergo regular antenatal check-ups for early detection of symptoms. Any other mild symptoms during pregnancy like burning micturition, increased frequency of urine, persistent cough, diarrhea, abdominal pain, vaginal discharge, etc should not be neglected and attended to promptly. Prompt investigations and treatment of the disease will go a long way to prevent the complications arising from the disease and fever in general.

Conclusion

Although it is evident that fever during pregnancy can impact the fetus, not much research has been done on this subject and this is a topic that requires further in depth study. Yet it cannot be denied that increased temperature during pregnancy can pose to be a high risk factor for the mother and child and should not be neglected/taken lightly. Prompt treatment no doubt helps in reducing the impact on the fetal development but as the old and very clichéd adage goes "Prevention is always better, far superior and any day more economical than cure".

REFERENCES

1. Tumalapalli Venkateswara Rao, Professor at Travancore Medical College, Kollam Kerala Published in: Health and Medicine, Technology

2. Denise J Jamieson, Regan N Theiler, Sonja A. Rasmussen. 'Emerging Infections and Pregnancy Emerging Infectious Diseases. 2006;12(11).

3. Park's Textbook of Preventive & Social Medicine, K. Park, 23rd edition.

4. John M Graham. 'Marshall J. Edwards: discoverer of maternal hyperthermia as a human teratogen. Birth Defects' Res. Part A Clin. Mol. Teratol.: 2005, 73(11);857–64.

5. J Cawdell-Smith, J Upfold, M Edwards, M Smith 'Neural tube and other developmental anomalies in the guinea pig following maternal hyperthermia during early neural tube development.' Teratog., Carcinog. Mutagen.: 1992, 12(1);1–9.

6. Andrew E Czeizel, Erzsébet H Puhó, Nándor Acs, Ferenc Bánhidy. 'Delineation of a multiple congenital abnormality syndrome in the offspring of pregnant women affected with high fever-related disorders: a population-based study.' Congenit Anom (Kyoto): 2008, 48(4);158–66.

7. OussenyZerbo, Ana-Maria Losif, Cheryl Walker, Sally Ozonoff, Robin L. Hansen and Irva Hertz-Picciotto. 'Is Maternal Influenza or Fever During Pregnancy Associated with Autism or Developmental Delays? Results from the CHARGE (Childhood Autism Risks from Genetics and Environment) Study.' Journal of Autism and Developmental Disorders, 2013, 43:25–33.

8. Maharaj, D. "Fever in Pregnancy." Antimicrobe—Infectious disease and antimicrobial agents.

3

Fetus and Fever

Saurabh Dani

Fever is defined as an elevation of body temperature above normal daily variation. The threshold for fever is generally considered to be maternal temperature ≥38 degrees C (≥100.4 degrees F) orally.

Fever occurs when the hypothalamic thermoregulatory center is reset at a higher temperature by "endogenous pyrogens" produced by specific host cells in response to infection, inflammation, injury, or antigenic challenge. These pyrogenic polypeptides include the cytokines interleukin (IL)-1 alpha and IL-1 beta, IL-6, tumor necrosis factor (TNF)-alpha and TNF-beta, and interferon alpha.[1,2]

Maternal fever is a considerable common problem. Although maternal fever has been implicated as a human teratogen in several studies, no prospective study has adequately addressed the full spectrum of birth outcomes following such exposure in pregnancy.[3] The primary localization of the primary infection significantly affects the impact of maternal fever on fetal behavior.[4]

Effect of maternal fever on fetus can be broadly classified in two categories:
1. Structural problems
2. Functional problems

Maternal fever resulting in preterm delivery has significant effect on the fetal outcome. About 25% of preterm deliveries are due to maternal infection/inflammation causing fever. The effects of preterm are seen in a neonate and not fetus and hence aptly shall not be discussed here.

How does Maternal Fever affect the fetus?

The effects of maternal fever on fetus is either due to the hyperthermia itself or the infection that causes it.

Maternal hyperthermia may result in the damage to the extraembryonic membranes, placenta, and maternal-fetal circulation, resulting in growth retardation, malformations, and fetal demise, and in the longer-term, to impaired cognitive function.

Common classes of problems associated with maternal fever are:
1. Neural tube defects
2. Congenital heart defects
3. Oral clefts
4. Limb deficiencies
5. Renal defects
6. Anorectal malformation
7. Ear defects
8. Cataracts
9. Allergic diseases

There is a 1.5 to 3 fold increase in neural tube defects, congenital heart defects and oral clefts when fetus is exposed to maternal fever in the first trimester.

Type of infection also determines the effect of maternal fever will have on fetus:

Infection	Significant effects on fetus
Malaria	Miscarriage, affects fetal growth
Typhoid	Fetal demise
Human Parovirus B19	Fetal anemia, non-immune fetal hydrops, fetal demise
CMV	Intracranial abnormalities
Rubella	Vision, hearing, brain defects, heart defects
Chorioamnionitis	Preterm labor, PROM

FUNCTIONAL DEFECTS IN FETUS

Detecting neurological disorders inutero seems to be an immense challenge for modern obstetrics. The massive cost incurred on its treatment and its effect on the quality of life of the affected not forgetting the strain on the immediate family warrants attention to detect them in utero. Fetal behavior is a window to view the functional status of the fetal brain. Early identification of abnormal fetal behavior offers a hope for early diagnosis of fetal neurological impairment and therapy. KANET test could be a tool to identify behavioral problems in the fetus.

What is KANET test?

Kurjak's antenatal neurobehavioral test (KANET) is a new scoring system for fetal neurobehavior, that has been recently introduced and is based on prenatal assessment of the fetus by 3D/4D ultrasound.[5,6] This scoring system is a combination of some parameters consisting of fetal general movements (GM) and of postnatal Amiel-Tison Neurological Assessment at Term (ATNAT) signs, which can be easily visualized prenatally by using 4D ultrasound.[7,8] The parameters were chosen based on developmental approach to the neurological assessment and on the theory of central pattern generators of general movement semergence, and were the product of multicentric studies conducted for several years.[9,10] The KANET test was standardized in Osaka, Japan, in order for the test to become reproducible and easily applied by fetal

medicine specialists. According to the Osaka Consensus Statement the KANET should be performed in the 3rd trimester of pregnancy, between 28 and 38 weeks. The duration of the examination should be between 15–20 minutes, and fetuses should be examined while they are awake. If the fetus is in the sleeping period, the assessment should be postponed for 30 minutes or for the following day, at a minimum period of 14–16 hours.

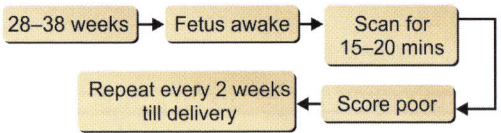

In cases of grossly abnormal or of borderline score, the test should be repeated every two weeks until delivery. Special attention should be paid to the facial movements and to eye blinking, which are prenatally very informative and important (the face is the mirror of the brain). The frequency of facial and mouth movements should be 0–5 and more than 5. Overall number of movements should be defined in very active or inactive fetuses and compared with normal values of previous studies.

The test evaluates quantitative as well as qualitative aspects of fetal motor behavioral patterns.

More recent studies show evidence that KANET is easily applicable to the majority of pregnancies, the learning curve is short for physicians who already have training in obstetrical ultrasound and the actual time of the KANET is very reasonable, ranging from 15–20 minutes, showing strong evidence that it can be widely implemented for fetal neurological assessment.[12]

As a conclusion, the results of recent, large multicenter studies show that KANET is an easily applied, standardized test, which utilizes the advantages of 4D ultrasound, such as better analysis of facial expressions and quality (variability and complexity) of fetal movements, in order to distinguish between normal and abnormal behavioral patterns of the fetus, with the aim of early recognition of fetal brain impairment.

ANTIPYRETIC MEDICATION

One of the most common treatments for maternal fever would be antipyretic medications. There is data to suggest that antipyretic medications may have a protective effect when used in relation to febrile episodes.[13,14,15]

Acetaminophen (which is a commonly used over-the-counter medication for fever) is a hormone disruptor, and abnormal hormonal exposures in pregnancy may influence fetal brain development. Maternal acetaminophen use during pregnancy is associated with a higher risk for HKDs and ADHD-like behaviors in children.[16]

REFERENCES

1. Smulian JC, B. V.-S.-L.(n.d.). Intrapartum fever at term: serum and histologic markers of inflammation. Am J Obstet Gynecol. 2003;188(1):269.
2. Saper CB, B. C. (n.d.). The neurologic basis of fever. N Engl J Med. 1994;330(26):1880.
3. Chambers CD, J. K. (n.d.). Maternal fever and birth outcome: A prospective study. Teratology. 1998 Dec;58(6):251–7.
4. Talic A, Kurjak A, Honemeyer U. Effect of Maternal Fever of Fetal Behaviour Assessed by KANET Test. Donald School J Ultrasound ObstetGynecol 2012;6(2): 160–165.
5. Systematic Review and Meta-analyses: Fever in Pregnancy and Health Impacts in the Offspring. Julie Werenberg Dreier, Anne-Marie Nybo Andersen, and Gabriele Berg-Beckhoff. Pediatrics peds.2013-3205; published ahead of print February 24, 2014, doi:10.1542/peds.2013–3205
6. Kurjak A, Miskovic B, Stanojevic M, Amiel-Tison C, Ahmed B, Azumendi G, Vasilj O, Andonotopo W, Turudic T, Salihagic-Kadic A. New scoring system for fetal neurobehavior assessed by three- and four-dimensional sonography. J Perinat Med. 2008;36(1):73–81.
7. Amiel-Tison C, Gosselin J, Kurjak A. Neuro-sonography in the second half of fetal life: a neonatologist's point of view. J Perinat Med. 2006;34(6):437–46.
8. Milan Stanojevic, Amira Talic, Berivoj Miskovic, Oliver Vasilj, Afaf Naim Shaddad, Badreldeen Ahmed, Aida Salihagic Kadic, Maja Predojevic, Radu Vladareanu, Daniela Lebit Salwa Abu-Yaqoub, Madeeha Al-Noobi. An Attempt to Standardize Kurjak's Antenatal Neurodevelopmental Test: Osaka Consensus Statement. DSJUOG. October–December 2011. Volume 5. pp 317–329.
9. Kurjak A, Andonotopo W, Hafner T, Salihagic Kadic A, Stanojevic M, Azumendi G, Ahmed B, Carrera JM, Troyano JM. Normal standards for fetal neurobehavioral developments— longitudinal quantification by four-dimensional sonography. J Perinat Med. 2006;34(1):56–65.
10. Kurjak A, Stanojevic M, Andonotopo W, Scazzocchio-Duenas E, Azumendi G, Carrera JM. Fetal behavior assessed in all three trimesters of normal pregnancy by four-dimensional ultrasonography. Croat Med J. 2005 Oct;46(5): 772–80.
11. Milan Stanojevic, Amira Talic, Berivoj Miskovic, Oliver Vasilj, Afaf Naim Shaddad, Badreldeen Ahmed, Aida Salihagic Kadic, Maja Predojevic, RaduVladareanu, Daniela Lebit Salwa Abu-Yaqoub, Madeeha Al-Noobi. An Attempt to Standardize Kurjak's Antenatal Neurodevelopmental Test: Osaka Consensus Statement. DSJUOG. October–December 2011. Volume 5, pp 317–329.
12. Miskovic B, Vasilj O, Stanojevic M, Ivankoviæ D, Kerner M, Tikvica A. The comparison of fetal behavior in high risk and normal pregnancies assessed by four dimensional ultrasound. J Matern Fetal Neonatal Med. 2010 Dec;23(12): 1461–7.
13. Czeizel AE, Puhó EH, Acs N, Bánhidy F. High fever-related maternal diseases as possible causes of multiple congenital abnormalities: a population-based case-control study. Birth Defects Res A ClinMolTeratol.2007;79(7):544–551.
14. Suarez L, Felkner M, Hendricks K. The effect of fever, febrile illnesses, and heat exposures on the risk of neural tube defects in a Texas-Mexico border population. Birth Defects Res A ClinMolTeratol. 2004;70(10):815–819.
15. Abe K, Honein MA, Moore CA. Maternal febrile illnesses, medication use, and the risk of congenital renal anomalies. Birth Defects Res A ClinMolTeratol. 2003;67(11):911–918.
16. Liew Z, Ritz B, Rebordosa C, Lee PC, Olsen J. Acetaminophen use during pregnancy, behavioral problems, and hyperkinetic disorders. JAMA Pediatr. 2014 Apr;168(4):313–20. doi: 10.1001/jamapediatrics.2013.4914.

4

Immunization in Pregnancy

Anahita Chauhan, Madhva Prasad

INTRODUCTION AND BACKGROUND

Infectious diseases continue to be a major cause of morbidity during pregnancy in all parts of the world, especially the developing countries. Susceptibility, duration or severity of morbidity of these diseases may increase during pregnancy. While other parts of this book deal with the management of such morbidities, this chapter is dedicated to vaccination against these diseases.

Ever since their introduction, there has been an ever expanding repertoire of vaccines available. The importance of appropriate nutrition and general healthcare measures in pregnancy has always received attention; vaccination as a specific cost effective health intervention which the obstetrician should offer all patients, has hitherto been neglected especially in our country. By and large, the obstetrician is only attuned to administering tetanus toxoid (TT). In this context, it is important to understand the available options, recommendations and new evidence for vaccination of pregnant and postpartum women.

Traditionally, immunization has been considered to be the prerogative of pediatricians and physicians. Pregnant women are at risk for vaccine-preventable disease-related morbidity and mortality and adverse pregnancy outcomes, such as congenital anomalies, abortions, prematurity and low birth weight. Apart from providing direct maternal benefit, vaccination during pregnancy also provides direct fetal and neonatal benefit through passive immunity (trans-placental transfer of maternal antibodies induced by vaccination).[1, 2]

Vaccination is the administration of antigenic material to stimulate an individual's immune system to develop adaptive immunity to a pathogen. Immunizations against specific infectious diseases protect individuals from symptomatic illnesses, blunt the severity of clinical illness, reduce complications and/or reduce transmission of infectious disease. Special situations such as travel to endemic areas would also necessitate vaccination.[3]

Vaccines, in general, work in the principle that the benefit of vaccination is usually greater than the potential risk when the possibility of exposure to that particular infection is high. In the context of pregnancy, benefit to the neonate should also be a consideration.

GENERAL GUIDELINES FOR IMMUNIZATION IN PREGNANCY

The Advisory Committee on Immunization Practices (ACIP) of the Centers for Disease Control (CDC), USA has recommended guidelines for vaccination in pregnancy:[4]

- As a general guideline, vaccination history should be elicited in all women in the reproductive age, and the possibility of pregnancy should be considered prior to any vaccination.

- Immunization history should be taken at first antenatal visit.
- All live viral vaccines as a rule are contraindicated during pregnancy; however, this risk is largely theoretical. Inactivated viral and bacterial vaccines and toxoids are safe in pregnancy.
- Benefits of vaccinating pregnant women usually outweigh potential risks when
  - The likelihood of disease exposure is high
  - When infection would pose a risk to the mother or fetus
  - When the vaccine is unlikely to cause harm
- Women who have inadvertently received live vaccine during pregnancy should not be counseled to terminate the pregnancy for teratogenic risk.
- Non-pregnant women should delay pregnancy for at least 4 weeks (this is a change in the previous recommendation of 3 months).
- Inactivated viral vaccines, bacterial vaccines and toxoids are safe.
- Breast feeding women can be immunized safely.

TETANUS TOXOID (TT) AND TETANUS DIPHTHERIA (TD)

Two doses of tetanus toxoid injection at least 28 days' apart should be given to all pregnant mothers commencing from second trimester. If the subsequent pregnancy occurs within 5 years only one booster is given.[5]

Both tetanus and diphtheria toxoids (Td) and TT vaccines have been used extensively in pregnant women worldwide to prevent neonatal tetanus; their administration has not been shown to be teratogenic. Current recommendation is that everyone should be given a booster shot for tetanus and diphtheria every 10 years after first being immunized;

hence Td during pregnancy has replaced TT in many parts of the world.

WHO recommends that for women who have not been previously immunized or whose immunization status is unknown, 2 doses of TT or Td during pregnancy, one month apart, with the second dose at least 2 weeks' prior to delivery affords protection during pregnancy. If the woman has received 1 to 4 TT doses in the past, give only 1 dose of TT or Td during pregnancy as a total of 5 doses protects during her childbearing years.[5]

Tdap [**T**etanus (T), **d**iphtheria (d) and **a**cellular **p**ertussis (ap)]

Scope of the Problem

Pertussis is a highly contagious respiratory infection caused by *Bordetella pertussis* which colonizes the respiratory tract mucous membranes and produces toxins that damage mucosa and induce systemic effects; the typical spasms of coughing end with a "whoop". Both the incidence and mortality are underestimated and underreported. Despite generally high coverage with childhood pertussis vaccines, it is one of the leading causes of deaths worldwide. Childhood vaccination does not confer lifelong immunity; this wanes after 4–12 years. Most deaths occur in young infants who are either unvaccinated or incompletely vaccinated. There have been increasing reports of cases in older children and adults, with adolescents and adults (especially parents) being a significant reservoir of infection for unvaccinated/partially vaccinated infants.

In recent years, a decrease in diphtheria–pertussis–tetanus (DPT) vaccine compliance has also been reported from different parts of India.[6, 7]

Rationale of Tdap Vaccination in Pregnancy

"Cocooning" is the strategy of vaccinating parents, siblings, grandparents, and health workers who are likely to have close contact with an infant aged < 12 months. These contacts, especially pregnant women in the later part of pregnancy or immediately postpartum should receive Tdap to reduce the risk for transmission of pertussis to infants, ideally at least 2 weeks prior to the anticipated contact. Tdap is a combination inactive vaccine that contains tetanus (T), diphtheria (d) and acellular pertussis (ap) in a single injection, and provides protection against all three; it is approved for adolescents from the age of 11 (younger contacts should receive DTaP) and adults ages 19 to 64. There is no live vaccine component in Tdap; it is manufactured using inactivated non-infectious bacterial products that generate a robust immune response. Some studies have suggested that maternal antibodies to pertussis can inhibit production of active pertussis-specific antibody after administration of DTaP vaccine to infants of mothers vaccinated with Tdap during pregnancy, referred to as "blunting". However, the benefit of protection given by maternal antibodies in newborn infants is much higher than the risk of shifting the burden of the disease to later in infancy.

Dosage

The recommended dose is one injection of Tdap during each pregnancy irrespective of the patient's prior history of receiving Tdap. Although Tdap may be given at any time during pregnancy, the ideal time for administration is between 27 and 36 weeks of gestation, which maximizes the maternal antibody response and transfer of antibodies to the neonate. Hence ideally the first dose of TT should be replaced with Td and the second, with Tdap. If Tdap is not administered during pregnancy, it should be administered soon after delivery. Along with several international agencies like Advisory Committee on Immunization Practices (ACIP) of CDC, Indian Academy of Pediatricians

(IAP) in their 2013 guidelines and FOGSI in their 2014 guidelines also strongly recommend Tdap to pregnant women. [2, 4, 8, 9,10]

From a safety perspective, ACIP concluded that administration of Tdap after 20 weeks' gestation is preferred to minimize the risk for any low-frequency adverse event and the possibility that any spurious association might appear causative.

INFLUENZA

Influenza is a highly contagious acute respiratory illness caused by infection with influenza viruses (Orthomyxoviridae) which affects the upper and lower respiratory tracts and produces systemic signs and symptoms. Three types, Influenza A, B and C, are determined by their nuclear material; influenza A subtypes are further divided based on H and N surface glycoproteins. "Flu" is often mistaken for the common cold, but has serious and far reaching complications. Global pandemics and epidemics cause a huge disease burden; though pregnancy does not increase susceptibility to influenza infection, pregnant women in the second and third trimesters of pregnancy are at increased risk for hospitalization, severe illness, serious complications like pneumonia and death. Mothers are increased risk of serious morbidity like especially preeclampsia and preterm labor; low birth weight, lower Apgar scores at birth and stillbirth has also been reported. It is critical to vaccinate against influenza before the season begins; however, this cannot be predicted accurately due to geographical and other variations. Hence international bodies recommend routine influenza vaccination for all women who are or will be pregnant (in any trimester) during influenza season. In case of outbreaks of influenza prior to the season, vaccination should be given to all pregnant women. A single dose of the trivalent inactivated vaccine (TIV) intramuscularly is recommended; the live attenuated nasal spray is contraindicated in pregnancy. Immunization to the mother affords protection to the infant for at least the first 6 months of life. ACOG guidelines state that "preventing influenza during pregnancy is an essential element of prenatal care, and the most effective strategy for preventing influenza is annual immunization". This is endorsed by many other agencies including WHO, ACIP (CDC) and Indian Academy of Pediatrics (IAP). FOGSI also recommends the vaccine after 26 weeks' gestation. [2, 11, 12, 13]

HEPATITIS B

Hepatitis B poses a serious risk to infants at birth and universal screening with HBsAg for all pregnant women is recommended. Pregnant women who are considered as being at risk of developing HBV infection during pregnancy (more than one sex partner during the preceding 6 months, evaluated or treated for an STI, recent or current intravenous drug abuse, or an HBsAg-positive sex partner) should be tested with antibody to surface antigen (anti-HBs) and be vaccinated if negative. Vaccination should be given only if clearly needed and possible advantages outweigh the possible risks. There are limited data which suggest that developing fetuses are not at risk for adverse events following hepatitis B vaccine. Babies should get HBIG at birth and first dose of vaccine within 12 hours of life. However, it is to be noted that no RCTs are available to give any specific recommendation at present. [4, 10, 14, 15]

HEPATITIS A

Though the safety of hepatitis A vaccination during pregnancy has not been determined, the theoretical risk to the developing fetus is expected to be low. Because hepatitis A vaccine is produced from inactivated hepatitis A virus (HAV), it is recommended during pregnancy only when the pregnant woman might be at high risk for exposure to HAV, including travel to endemic areas. [3, 4, 10]

MEASLES-MUMPS-RUBELLA (MMR) VACCINE

Specifically due to the adverse effects of rubella on the fetus, the MMR vaccine and its component vaccines should not be administered to women known to be pregnant or attempting to conceive. Because of the theoretical risk to the fetus when the mother receives a live viral vaccine, women should be counseled to avoid becoming pregnant for 28 days after receipt of the vaccine. The previous recommendations suggesting avoidance of pregnancy for 3 months have been revised. [4, 10]

VARICELLA

Since the effects of varicella infection on the fetus are not known, immunization is not recommended. However, if there is documented exposure to varicella, passive immunization in the form of varicella zoster immunoglobulin is recommended. [4, 10]

MENINGOCOCCAL VACCINE

Along the spectrum of presentations of meningococcal infections are pneumonia, meningitis and meningococcal septicemia, which can occur sporadically or as outbreaks. ACIP and the WHO recommend that for both meningococcal conjugate (MCV4/Men ACWY) and meningococcal polysaccharide (MPSV4), both inactivated bacterial vaccines, pregnancy should not preclude vaccination, if indicated. [3, 4, 10, 16]

POLIOMYELITIS

The polio eradication programme has made significant strides and India has now been declared polio free; hence in the current Indian context, polio vaccine is not considered for adults. [4, 10]

PNEUMOCOCCUS

ACIP recommends that the inactivated bacterial vaccine of pneumococcal polysaccharide (PPSV23) may be considered for routine vaccination. Though no adverse consequences have been reported among newborns whose mothers were inadvertently vaccinated during pregnancy, it has not been fully evaluated in the first trimester.[3, 4, 10]

HUMAN PAPILLOMAVIRUS (HPV)

HPV vaccines are not recommended for use in pregnant women. If a woman is found to be pregnant after initiating the vaccination series, the remainder of the three-dose series should be delayed until completion of pregnancy. However, if a vaccine dose has been administered during pregnancy, no intervention or termination of pregnancy is warranted. [4, 8, 10]

RABIES

As post-exposure prophylaxis is vital due to the potential consequences of inadequately managed rabies exposure, pregnancy is not considered a contraindication. It may be recommended routinely to those who are particularly at high risk for exposure, e.g. those handling animals. [4, 10]

JAPANESE ENCEPHALITIS AND YELLOW FEVER

These viral diseases can have significant morbidity, especially when contracted during pregnancy. These vaccines should be considered only when the potential risk of infection is high, or during unavoidable travel to an endemic area with high infection rate during pregnancy. [3, 4, 10]

ANTHRAX

Vaccination is considered only in the post-event setting. If the woman is at significant risk, anthrax adsorbed vaccine is recommended along with antimicrobial prophylaxis.[10]

Summary of recommendations (modified from CDC ACIP guidelines 2012)[4]				
Vaccine	Before Pregnancy	During Pregnancy	After Pregnancy	Type of vaccine
Hepatitis A	Yes if indicated	Yes if indicated	Yes if indicated	Inactivated
Hepatitis B	Yes if indicated	Yes if indicated (high risk patients)	Yes if indicated	Inactivated
Human papillo-mavirus (HPV)	Yes	No	Yes	Inactivated
Influenza TIV	Yes	Yes	Yes	Inactivated
Influenza live attenuated	Yes if indicated Avoid conception for 4 weeks	No	Yes if indicated	Live
MMR	Yes, if indicated. Avoid conception for 4 weeks	No	Yes, if indicated. Give immediately post-partum, if susceptible to rubella	Live
Tdap	Yes, if indicated	Yes, vaccinate during each pregnancy ideally between 27 and 36 weeks of gestation	Yes, immediately post-partum, if not received previously	Toxoid/ inactivated
Tetanus/ Diphtheria Td	Yes, if indicated	Yes, if indicated. Tdap preferred	Yes, if indicated	Toxoid
Varicella	Yes, if indicated, avoid conception for 4 weeks	No	Yes, if indicated. Give immediately postpartum, if susceptible	Live

TYPHOID, HEMOPHILUS AND BCG

At present no prospective studies and no current recommendations exist for use of typhoid and *Hemophilus influenzae* B vaccines in pregnancy. Bacillus Calmette Guérin (BCG) vaccine is not recommended for use in pregnant women.

POSTPARTUM VACCINATION

The puerperal period is an excellent window of opportunity for vaccination of women and promotion of positive health advice. It is safe for a woman to receive routine vaccines after birth and in the lactation period. A woman who has not received Tdap or influenza vaccine should be vaccinated right after delivery and a woman who is not immune to measles, mumps and rubella and/or varicella (chickenpox) should be vaccinated before she leaves the hospital. HPV vaccine is also safe during the lactation period.[4]

CONCLUSIONS

In conclusion, maternal vaccination is a cost-effective and targeted strategy to improve pregnancy outcomes in developed and developing countries. Many national organizations have followed the lead of international public health agencies, and recommend vaccination during pregnancy for influenza and Tdap; obstetricians should now include these as a part of the routine immunization schedule. Lack of awareness of benefits and concerns about vaccine safety in pregnancy, both in the minds of the provider and the patient, are common barriers to vaccination.

REFERENCES

1. Swamy GK, Heine RP. Vaccinations for pregnant women. Obstet Gynec 2015 Jan; 125(1):212–26.

2. AR Chauhan. Vaccination in pregnancy. Editorial. J Postgrad Gyn Obs. Mar 2015: 2 (3). Available at http://www.jpgo.org/2015/03/editorial.html. Last accessed 8th June 2015.

3. Jackson LA, Schuchat A. Immunization Principles and Vaccine Use *In:* Longo DL, Kasper DL, Jameson JL , Fauci AS, Hauser SL, Loscalzo J, editors. Harrison's principles of internal medicine,18th ed., McGraw-Hill; 2012.

4. Rasmussen SA, Watson AK, Kennedy ED, Broder KR, Jamieson DJ. Vaccines and pregnancy: Past, present, and future. ACIP recommendations. Seminars in Fetal & Neonatal Medicine: 19 (2014): 161–169.

5. Maternal Immunization against Tetanus. Integrated management of pregnancy and childbirth. WHO publication. Available at www.who.in/reproductivehealth/publications/maternal_perinatal_health/immunization_tetanus.pdf. Last accessed 8th June, 2015.

6. Amrithalingam G, Andrews N, Campbell H, Ribeiro S, Kara E, Donegan K et al. Effectiveness of maternal pertussis vaccination in England: an observational study. Lancet. 2014 Oct 25;384 (9953):1521–8.

7. Centers for Disease Prevention and Control. Pertussis surveillance and reporting http://www.cdc.gov/pertussis/surv-reporting/cases-by-year.html. Last accessed 29th April 2015.

8. Pandit SN et al. Vaccination in Women. FOGSI Consensus Statement. September 2014.

9. Centers for Disease Control and Prevention. Updated Recommendations for Use of Tetanus Toxoid, Reduced Diphtheria Toxoid and Acellular Pertussis Vaccine (Tdap) in Pregnant Women and Persons Who Have or Anticipate Having Close Contact with an Infant Aged <12 Months — Advisory Committee on Immunization Practices (ACIP), 2011. MMWR 2011; 60:41 [1424].

10. Sharma RK, Ruhela V. Immunization in Pregnant Women *In :* Muruganathan A, Mathai D, Sharma SK, Eds. Adult Immunisation.1st ed. Jaypee; 2014.

11. Vashishtha VM, Kalra A and Choudhury P. Influenza Vaccination in India: Position Paper of Indian Academy of Pediatrics. Indian Pediatrics. Sept 2013; 50(9): 867–874.

12. Centers for Disease Control and Prevention. Prevention and Control of Seasonal Influenza with Vaccine. Recommendations of the Advisory Committee on Immunization Practices. MMWR 2013; 62 (No.7): 30.

13. Influenza vaccination coverage among pregnant women: 2011–12 influenza season, United States. MMWR Morb Mortal Wkly Rep. 2012 Sep 28; 61: 758–63.

14. Mast EE, Weinbaum CM, Fiore AE, Alter MJ, Bell BP, Finelli L, et al. A comprehensive immunization strategy to eliminate transmission of hepatitis B virus infection in the United States: Recommendations of the Advisory Committee on Immunization Practices (ACIP). Part II: Immunization of adults. MMWR Recomm Rep 2006; 55:1e33

15. Sangkomkamhang US, Lumbiganon P, Laopaiboon M. Hepatitis B vaccination during pregnancy for preventing infant infection. Cochrane Database Syst Rev 2014 Nov 11;11: CD007879. doi: 10.1002/14651858. CD007879. pub3

16. Meningococcus Global Advisory Committee on Vaccine Safety, June 2014. Weekly epidemiological record No. 29, 2014, 89, 321–336. Available from: http://www.who.int/wer/2014/wer8929. pdf. Last accessed 8th July 2015.

5

Neonatal Issues

Sanjay B Prabhu

Hyperthermia, i.e. temperature above 103°F is not uncommon during pregnancy. The duration of fever and time of occurrence during gestation and the maximum temperature reached determine the fetal effects irrespective of the cause of the fever.

Prenatal death and abortion is seen in severe hyperthermia in the mother during embryonic and fetal development and mild elevations in temperature can cause the same in preimplantation period. A wide range of structural and functional defects especially of the central nervous system have been seen in the fetus due to hyperthermia especially in the first trimester.

In the largest ever epidemiologic study to examine effects of hyperthermia on the fetus, Dreier, et al have reported an elevated risk for poor health outcomes among children exposed to maternal fever in utero for three common classes of defects: Neural tube defects, congenital heart defects and oral clefts. The researchers identified 1.5 to nearly 3 fold increased risk with exposure during first trimester for 9 case control studies of neural tube defects, 5 case control studies of oral clefts and 7 studies for congenital heart defects. Other uncommon defects included limb deficiencies, renal defects, anorectal malformation, ear defects, cataracts, and allergic diseases. Some studies showed lowered risk with use of antipyretic medication.

The researchers conclude that they "found substantial evidence to support an adverse impact of maternal fever during pregnancy."

PHYSIOLOGY OF HYPERTHERMIA IN MOTHER AND EFFECTS ON THE FETUS

There are several mechanisms through which fever has been proposed to interfere with the fetal development. When infection in pregnancy occurs, the maternal immune system is mobilized, causing changes in the level of cytokines in the fetal environment. Some cytokines, such as interleukin 1, interleukin 6, and tumor necrosis factor, are pyrogenic, causing hyperthermia to occur through alteration of the set point in the hypothalamus. Hypothesized effects of the increased body temperature include interruption of protein synthesis and enzyme production. In addition, as a reaction to the fever, the heat shock response is induced. The response acts as a survival mechanism, and the expression of heat shock proteins is increased to enhance cellular resistance to thermal stress. The heat shock response takes precedence over other cellular activities, resulting in inhibition of protein synthesis and cell proliferation. It is consequently believed that these mechanisms may disturb or harm the fetal development if they coincide with specific windows of vulnerability. Exposures in middle and late pregnancy may lead to longer-term adverse effects in the child.

Nevertheless, the current evidence is insufficient to conclude whether fever might be harmful in all stages of pregnancy. It is well established that several infections, such as the TORCH complex have teratogenic effects. In addition, a range of other infections (e.g. influenza, Q fever, HIV) are suspected of having detrimental effects on the child but as of now these are unproven.

INFECTIONS AND PREGNANCY

1. Respiratory Infections

A. Chickenpox

80% of all pregnant women are found to be immune to chickenpox on testing though chickenpox during pregnancy has high incidence of pneumonia and mortality in the mother. Herpes zoster during pregnancy has no deleterious effects on the fetus.

The primary risk of maternal chickenpox in early pregnancy is fetal infection, which may result in the congenital varicella syndrome. In the first 20 weeks of pregnancy, the risk of embryopathy after maternal varicella infection is less than 2 percent. Congenital varicella syndrome is characterized by limb hypoplasia, cutaneous scarring, chorioretinitis, microphthalmia, Horner's syndrome, cataracts, cortical atrophy, mental retardation, microcephaly and low birth weight.

Maternal varicella infection between five days before and two days after delivery poses a substantial risk to the neonate. Neonatal varicella is a severe infection that manifests with skin lesions and pneumonia and has a mortality rate of up to 31 percent. In the first 10 days of life, up to 50 percent of these infants will be affected.

B. Fifth Disease

Fifth disease (erythema infectiosum) is caused by human parvovirus B19, a single-stranded DNA virus that affects only humans. The disease is transmitted through respiratory secretions and hand-to-mouth transfer.

Children with fifth disease present with a widespread, lacy, erythematous rash with malar flushing ("slapped cheeks"). Adults with fifth disease are less likely to develop the facial rash and are more likely to have arthralgias, although 20 percent of adults are asymptomatic. Current guidelines do not recommend exclusion from the workplace where fifth disease is present because of the low risk to the fetus.

Although human parvovirus B19 infections are not teratogenic, they can destroy erythroid precursors and cause fetal anemia, which may lead to subsequent heart failure, nonimmune hydrops and death. The rate of transplacental transmission is approximately 30 percent. When maternal infection occurs before 20 weeks of gestation, the rate of fetal loss is 9 percent.

C. Cytomegalovirus

It is the most common intrauterine infection seen in 1% of all pregnancies though it largely remains asymptomatic in mothers. Fever as a manifestation of CMV infection is rarely seen.

D. Influenza and the Common Cold

Influenza is generally self-limited in healthy young adults. However, if pneumonia develops, it can be life-threatening and may be more severe in pregnancy. WHO recommends influenza vaccine for all women who will be in the second or third trimester of pregnancy during the influenza season. Pregnant women, especially those with co-morbidities, are at increased risk for complications from all forms of influenza virus infection—seasonal, zoonotic, and pandemic (H1N1).

Influenza in pregnancy is associated with an increased risk of adverse pregnancy outcomes, such as spontaneous abortion, preterm birth, and fetal distress. Pregnant women appear to be approximately 4–5 times more likely to develop severe disease, when compared to non-pregnant individuals in the general population, and this risk is highest in the third trimester.

Concern has been raised about a possible association between influenza in early pregnancy and anencephaly, but there is no firm evidence that influenza adversely affects the fetus.

Influenza-specific antibody is transmitted to the fetus in utero and protects the newborn.

E. *Rubella*

Before the vaccine became available in 1969, congenital rubella was a major cause of malformations in neonates. While the vaccine has not caused malformations, it should be avoided during pregnancy and contraception should be used for three months after vaccination. The susceptible mother should be vaccinated in the immediate postpartum period, regardless of whether she plans to breast-feed.

The risk to the fetus varies with gestational age. Pregnant women who are exposed to rubella should have immediate serologic evaluation for IgG and IgM. If primary rubella is diagnosed in the first trimester of pregnancy, the patient should be counseled about the option to undergo termination of pregnancy. If IgG antibody is present at the time of exposure, the mother should be reassured that she is immune.

F. *Other Viruses*

Isolated reports of fetal malformation are associated with other respiratory viruses. However, the lack of consistent patterns justifies reassurance for mothers who have been exposed to measles, mumps, adenoviruses, respiratory syncytial virus (bronchiolitis), Epstein-Barr virus (infectious mononucleosis) and human herpesvirus 6 (roseola). First-trimester infection with mumps or human herpesvirus 6 may increase the risk of spontaneous abortion, but an increase in the risk from measles, infectious mononucleosis or respiratory syncytial virus has not been documented.

2. Malaria in Pregnancy

Malaria infection during pregnancy is a significant public health problem with substantial risks for the pregnant woman, her fetus, and the newborn child. Malaria-associated maternal illness and low birth weight is mostly the result of *Plasmodium falciparum* infection and occurs predominantly in Africa.

The symptoms and complications of malaria in pregnancy vary according to malaria transmission intensity in the given geographical area, and the individual's level of acquired immunity.

In high-transmission settings, where levels of acquired immunity tend to be high, *P. falciparum* infection is usually asymptomatic in pregnancy. Yet, parasites may be present in the placenta and contribute to maternal anaemia even in the absence of documented peripheral parasitaemia. Both maternal anaemia and placental parasitaemia can lead to low birth weight, which is an important contributor to infant mortality. In high-transmission settings, the adverse effects of *P. falciparum* infection in pregnancy are most pronounced for women in their first pregnancy.

In low-transmission settings, where women of reproductive age have relatively a little acquired immunity to malaria, malaria in pregnancy is associated with anaemia, an increased risk of severe malaria, and it may lead to spontaneous abortion, stillbirth, prematurity and low birth weight. In such settings, malaria affects all pregnant women, regardless of the number of times they have been pregnant.

Infection with *P. vivax*, as with *P. falciparum*, leads to chronic anaemia and placental malaria infection, reducing the birth weight and increasing the risk of neonatal death. For women in their first pregnancy, the reduction in birth weight is approximately two-thirds of what is associated with *P. falciparum*, but with *P. vivax* the effect appears to increase with successive pregnancies.

3. Dengue

Symptomatic dengue infection during pregnancy may increase the risk of Preterm birth and LBW for infants. More research is needed to confirm these results and to examine the role of dengue fever in abortions. Neonatal dengue is a rare possibility, if mother gets dengue fever just prior to delivery which allows the virus to transplacentally cross over.

4. Typhoid Fever

Typhoid fever is well-recognized endemic disease in our country. *Salmonella typhi* causes septicemia of digestive origin that can cross the placenta resulting in chorioamniotitis. Maternal-fetal infection with *S. typhi* can lead to miscarriage, fetal death, neonatal infection, as well as diverse maternal complications. In order to avoid maternal complications and possible fetal transmission, treatment with ceftriaxone should be initiated as early as possible.

5. Hepatitis in Pregnancy

Acute viral hepatitis is the most common cause of jaundice in pregnancy. The course of most viral hepatitis infections (e.g. hepatitis A, B, C and D) is unaffected by pregnancy, however, a more severe course of viral hepatitis in pregnancy has been observed in patients with hepatitis E. Notwithstanding, opinions differ over the maternal and fetal outcome of pregnancy associated with viral hepatitis. While some authors reported that acute viral hepatitis carries a high risk for both mother and fetus, others conclude that non-fulminant viral hepatitis did not influence the course of pregnancy or fetal well-being. Rate of transmission of the virus during pregnancy depends on the virus. For instance, intra-utero transmission of hepatitis A virus is very rare, but perinatal transmission could occur. Conversely sixty percent of pregnant women who acquire acute HBV infections at or near delivery will transmit the HBV virus to their offspring and mother to child transmission of hepatitis E virus infection was established between 33.3 and 50%. Breast-feeding is not contra-indicated in women infected with the hepatitis A, E or C. However, for acute hepatitis B, with appropriate immuno-prophylaxis, including hepatitis B immune globulin and hepatitis B vaccine, breast-feeding of infants of HBV infected mother's poses no additional risk for the transmission of the hepatitis B virus.

6. Chorioamnionitis

There is significant association between significant neurodevelopmental delay, cerebral palsy in the neonate and chorio-amnionitis especially when occuring just near term or extremely preterm births.

Intrauterine infection causes a fetal inflammatory response syndrome which is ignited due to high levels of inflammatory cytokines, tumor necrosis factor and chemokines leading to preterm labour, intrauterine growth restriction, cerebral ischemia and intraventricular hemorrhage and also leading to chronic lung disease in the neonate.

The most dreaded complication in the neonate is severe early onset neonatal sepsis going into septic shock and DIC and multi-organ dysfunction.

7. Intrapartum Fever

The most common infectious etiologies are intra-amniotic infection, urinary tract infection and respiratory infection in the mother and the most common non-infectious etiology being the use of epidural analgesia.

Maternal fever may have fetal/neonatal consequences even when infection is not cause of the fever. These children are seen to be hypotonic at birth with low apgar requiring resuscitation and may develop neonatal seizures.

8. HIV and Tuberculosis

These may present together or separately in a pregnant mother. HIV per se does not affect the fetus but transmission can occur during perinatal period and during breastfeeding, so measures should be taken to prevent this.

Tuberculosis if untreated or if it is the multidrug resistant variety may cause severe growth restriction, premature delivery or still-birth.

NONINFECTIOUS CAUSES OF FEVER IN PREGNANCY

There is scant literature on this subject except for a few case reports of such causes of fever and effect on the fetus.

CONCLUSION

Fever in pregnancy can have grave consequences for both mother and child and early diagnosis and prompt treatment is mandatory.

BIBLIOGRAPHY

1. Dreier JW, Systematic review and meta-analyses: Fever in pregnancy and health impact in the offspring. Pediatrics; 2014:133(3):e674–688.

Key messages

1. Prompt symptomatic treatment of fever in pregnancy vital.
2. Avoid and treat hyperthermia aggressively as it is detrimental to the fetus.
3. USG follow up of fetus exposed to hyperthermia in the first trimester mandatory.
4. Algorithms required to diagnose and manage fever in pregnancy
5. Neonatal follow up in high risk cases required for a period beyond infancy.

2. Ely JW, Evaluation of pregnant women exposed to respiratory viruses. AAFP;2000:0515: p3065html

3. WHO Fact Sheets on Influenza and Malaria in pregnancy.

4. Edwards MJ: Hyperthermia and fever during pregnancy. Birth Defects Part A:clinical and molecular teratology 2006;76(7):507–516.

5. Sookooian S, Liver disease in pregnancy:acute viral hepatitis. Annals of Hepatology 2006;5.

6. Lieberman E Intrapartum fever and neonatal outcome. Pediatrics 2000;105:8.

7. Cornette L. Fetal and Neonatal inflammatory response and adverse outcome. Seminars in Neonatal Medicine 2004;9:459.

8. Wu YW. Chorioamnionitis and cerbral palsy in term and near term infants. JAMA2003;290:2677.

Drugs in Pregnancy and Lactation

Shruti Bangale Daflapurkar

INTRODUCTION

Prescribing drugs in pregnant and lactating women is challenging for the clinician, who has to carefully balance effectively between treating the disease condition and limiting exposure to maternal drugs by the foetus or breastfeeding infant.

The awareness of the potential harm of drug use during pregnancy began a few decades ago, when the teratogenic effects of thalidomide were first recognized. Prior to this, there was a belief among clinicians and patients that developing embryos and foetuses were protected in utero from harmful effects of drugs by a "placental barrier".[1]

The placental barrier was believed to protect the fetus from substances taken by the mother similar to the blood–brain barrier. The concept of a placental barrier has now been abandoned. It is understood that the placenta only controls extent to and rate at which the medicine can reach to the foetus.

The drugs that are lipid soluble, have a high pH, or have a low molecular weight cross the placenta more readily. But, it must be considered that any drug absorbed through oral ingestion can potentially enter the fetal circulation.

Despite this recognition of fetal susceptibility to adverse effects of drugs, still, prescription drugs continue to be widely used during pregnancy. An international investigation sponsored by the World Health Organization showed that pregnant women ingest an average of three prescription medications during pregnancy.[2] This study has not included the use of over-the-counter drugs. There is a general tendency to have a pill for every symptom. This may partially explain the widespread use of drugs during pregnancy. However, the potential for adverse fetal effects suggests that casual use of drugs in pregnancy should be discouraged, particularly if the drug is being used to treat symptoms that are benign or self-limited.

There is a paradox as well. There is a tendency for both patients and clinicians to withhold needed treatments because of fear of foetal effects. This may be true even when the drug is required to manage serious maternal disease. Clinicians may tell pregnant women to discontinue important drugs, and patients often refuse needed medications—even when reasonable data support their use.

PATHOPHYSIOLOGY

Drugs can be harmful to the unborn baby because:
1. Drugs pass placenta by passive diffusion through lipid barrier between maternal and embryonic circulation
2. Non-ionised drugs pass more rapidly
3. Most drugs are small enough to pass with exceptions like growth hormones, conjugated steroids

EFFECTS OF DRUGS USE IN PREGNANCY

Drugs that can cause development of congenital malformations or other negative fetal outcomes are called teratogens. It includes:

1. Altered growth or development
2. Structural malformations
3. Physiological malformations
4. Mortality

Although teratogen exposure increases the risk of negative fetal outcomes, it does not ensure the occurrence of any fetal effects.

The probability of teratogen exposure will result in a negative outcome depends on several factors.

1. Drug dosage and duration of exposure
2. Gestational age during exposure
3. Individual susceptibility to exposure
4. Cumulative teratogenic exposures

Risk of a negative outcome is greater with higher drug dosages and longer duration of exposure. It increases with the additional use of other teratogenic agents or if the mother or baby is genetically more susceptible to development of a specific malformation or other negative outcome.

EFFECTS OF DRUGS IN PREGNANCY ACCORDING TO GESTATIONAL AGE

Preimplantation Period (Day 1–Day 7)

Damage of fertilized oocyte either leads to death or complete recovery. Contact with toxic chemicals or irradiation does not increase the risk of congenital malformations.

The First Trimester (Day 8–End of month 2)

This is the most important period for teratogenicity as this is the main period of organ formation.

3–9 Months

This is the period with less risk of teratogenicity except urogenital system and central nervous system. During this period there are more functional effects like bleeding with the use of salicylates and anticoagulant use increase the risk of bleeding.

Delivery

During this period drugs have effects in newborn, e.g. CNS depressants cause "Floppy baby syndrome", drugs with increased bleeding risk like salicylates and anticoagulants cause increased risk of cerebral hemorrhage in babies during delivery.

Medications Prescription during Pregnancy

The vast majority of pregnant women consume both prescription and non-prescription medications. In one survey, 578 obstetric patients were interviewed about their medication use.[3] Prescription medications (excluding vitamin, mineral, and iron supplements) were used by 60% of women, over-the-counter medications by 93%, and herbal remedies by 45%.

The four most commonly prescribed categories of medications were:
- Antibiotics (used by 35% of patients)
- Respiratory drugs (15%)
- Gastrointestinal products (13%)
- Opioids (8%)

The most commonly used over-the-counter drugs were analgesics like acetaminophen (76%), ibuprofen (15%), and aspirin (2%). Herbal remedies were usually peppermint for nausea (18%) and cranberry for urinary tract symptoms (13%).

Clinicians may be unaware that their patients are using over-the-counter therapies or prescriptions from other providers. Hence, they need to ask patients specifically about all prescription and non-prescription medications they are using.

Clinicians must be able to provide patients with credible information about safe treatment, as unfounded patient fears can result in substantial maternal stress and anxiety and even consideration of pregnancy termination.

A negative impact on pregnancy by maternal stress has been supported by studies showing that women exposed to high stress during pregnancy have a higher risk of delivering offspring with low birth weight when babies are born prematurely and a higher incidence of cranial-neural crest malformations [especially cleft lip/palate and conotruncal heart defects (e.g., double-outlet ventricle, tetralogy of Fallot, and ventricular septal defects)].[4, 5.]

Providing accurate information about safe treatment options can alleviate a considerable amount of the pregnant patient's fear and concern.

THINGS TO BE CONSIDERED BEFORE PRESCRIBING THE MEDICATION

1. Necessity of the Medication

Is the symptom self-limited or amenable to non-pharmacologic management?

Medication use in pregnancy has to be considered in terms of the necessity of the drug and the availability of alternatives. No drug should be used in pregnancy without a justifiable indication. For example, there is a good data which suggest safety of oral antifungal during pregnancy. But one should always wait to treat onychomycosis as it can be safely treated later.

Self-limited symptoms may require only reassurance from the clinician. If available, non-pharmacologic alternatives should be considered.

2. Necessity of the Treatment

A. Epilepsy in Pregnancy

It may be potentially dangerous to withhold certain important medications during pregnancy even though it may be harmful to the foetus. For example, although use of the anticonvulsant phenytoin during pregnancy doubles the risk of foetal malformations, experience has shown that uncontrolled seizures present a greater risk to mother and child.[6]

AED use can increase risk of malformation of almost all organs. The commonest malformations are orofacial clefts (cleft lip, cleft palate), congenital heart disease and neural tube defects. Among commonly used AEDs, valproic acid is associated with highest risk of malformations (8.6–16.7%), followed by phenytoin (3.4–10.5%), phenobarbitone (4.7–6.5%) and carbamazepine (2–5.2%). The risk of malformation is increased when the fetus is exposed to AEDs in the first trimester and when the AEDs are used in high doses.

It is advised that all pregnant with epilepsy should undergo fetal monitoring using maternal serum alpha-fetoprotein (MSAFP) at 16 weeks and a detailed ultrasonography screening at 18 weeks by an experienced sonographer to detect fetal malformations.

B. Tuberculosis in Pregnancy

Same argument can be put forth for use of anti-tuberculous drugs in pregnancy.

Isoniazide (INH): INH is safe during pregnancy even in the first trimester, though it can cross the placenta. Pyridoxine supplementation is recommended for all pregnant women taking INH at a dose of 50 mg daily.

Rifampicin: It is also believed to be safe in pregnancy, though in some cases, there is an increased risk of haemorrhagic disorders in the newborn. It can be prevented by giving supplemental vitamin K (10 mg/day) for the last four to eight weeks of pregnancy.

Ethambutol: The retrobulbar neuritis with this drug seen in adults generated the fear that it may interfere with ophthalmological development when used in pregnancy but this has not been demonstrated when the standard dose is used.

Pyrazinamide: There are no reports of significant adverse events from the use of this drug in the treatment of TB in pregnant women. Its use in pregnancy is recommended by WHO and RNTCP. It is particularly indicated in women with tuberculous meningitis in pregnancy, HIV co-infection and suspected INH resistance.

Streptomycin: The drug has been proven to be potentially teratogenic throughout pregnancy. It causes fetal malformations and eighth-nerve paralysis, with deficits ranging from mild hearing loss to bilateral deafness.

Pregnant MDR-TB: Standardized treatment regimen for the treatment of MDRTB is intensive phase which consists of 6–9 months of kanamycin, ofloxacin, ethionamide, cycloserine, pyrazinamide and ethambutol and continuation phase which consists of 18 months of ofloxacin, ethionamide, cycloserine and ethambutol.

Management of MDR-TB patients are based on the duration of pregnancy. For patients who are unwilling for MTP or have pregnancy of > 20 weeks, the risk to the mother and fetus needs to be explained clearly and a modified Cat IV should be started. For patients in the first trimester (≤ 12 weeks), kanamycin and Ethionamide are omitted from the Cat IV regimen and PAS is added. For patients who have completed the first trimester (>12 weeks), kanamycin is replaced with PAS. Post partum, PAS may be replaced with kanamycin and continued until the end of the intensive phase.

C. HIV in Pregnancy

Antiretroviral therapy should be offered to all pregnant women infected with HIV to reduce the risk of perinatal transmission. Zidovudine (ZDV) is the only agent specifically shown to reduce perinatal transmission, it should be used whenever possible as part of the highly active antiretroviral therapy (HAART) regimen.

If a patient who is on a HAART regimen presents for prenatal care, continuing her treatment during the first trimester is reasonable, provided that care is taken to avoid medications that are contraindicated in early pregnancy.

In an HIV-infected pregnant woman who has never been exposed to antiretroviral medication, HAART should be started as soon as possible, including during the first trimester.

If this test was performed on arrival in labor, treatment with the ZDV protocol through labor is recommended, followed by administration to the neonate until confirmatory testing on the mother becomes available.

Guidelines for perinatal ART were revised in July 2012 regarding which agents are considered preferred, alternative, or to be used under special circumstances. Combination regimens, usually including 2 NRTIs with either an NNRTI or 1 or more protease inhibitors (PIs) are recommended. For further information, see the Table below.

3. Justified use of Drugs in Pregnancy

1. High grade fever in the first few months of pregnancy is more harmful than use of paracetamol.
2. Diabetes in pregnancy requires monitoring and treatment with insulin.

ART agents during pregnancy			
Art class	Preferred	Alternate	Special circumstances
NRTIs	Zidovudine (AZT)	Abacavir	Didanosine
	Lamivudine (3TC)	Emtricitabine	Stavudine
		Tenofovir	
NNRTIs	Nevirapine	—	Efavirenz
PIs	Atazanavir Lopinavir +	Darunavir	Indinavir
	Ritonavir	Saquinavir	Nelfinavir
Integrase inhibitors	—	—	Raltegravir

4. Availability of Similar Drug with a Better Safety Profile

Very few medications have undergone rigorous studies to determine their effects on a developing human fetus. Most available safety information is derived from animal studies, retrospective analyses, case reports, and epidemiological data, all of which have significant limitations.

Post-marketing data obtained through pregnancy registries can also provide valuable information about pregnancy-related drug effects. But participation in these registries is voluntary, thus limiting data interpretation. Hence, no drug should be considered completely safe in pregnancy.

Clinicians should be more vigilant for drug safety during the first trimester of pregnancy, because it is during this time that organogenesis occurs and the developing embryo is at risk for teratogenesis. Hence, all efforts should be made during this period to avoid all unnecessary medications and any known teratogens. However, drugs taken at any time during gestation can affect the fetus. Medication toxicities and adverse effects on fetal neurologic development can occur during any trimester. Hence, the concept of "safe period" is never there. The fetus is never immune to potential drug effects.

Many drugs are identified as causing human embryologic or fetal toxicities only after they have been on the market for several years. Hence, as a general rule, clinicians prescribing drugs for pregnant women should have a bias toward older agents, because we have more clinical experience with their use in pregnancy.

5. Pharmacokinetic Changes in Pregnancy

Absorption

Slowed gastrointestinal motility can delay absorption of oral agents.

Renal Clearance

Glomerular filtration rates increase in pregnancy to 150% of normal range. Hence, many medications that are excreted through kidney require dosage alterations in pregnancy.

For example, digoxin doses may need to be increased to as much as 1mg by the end of the second trimester.

Hepatic Clearance

An increase in hepatic clearance of medicines is frequently seen during pregnancy.

Volume of Distribution

Plasma volume increases to 150% of normal by 24 to 28 weeks' gestation, increasing the volume of distribution. Hence, drugs may require dosage adjustments.

Protein Binding

Dilution of serum proteins—caused by the increase in free water that is responsible for most of the increase in blood volume during pregnancy—may lead to increased free drug levels for a particular total serum level.

The main practical applications of this information is dosing intervals may need to be shortened in pregnancy. Inadequate dosing frequency should always be considered as a possible cause for treatment failure. This is particularly true for once-a-day agents used to control hypertension; careful examination of blood pressure toward the end of a dosing interval may lead the clinician to increase dosing frequency. If required, medication levels should be periodically monitored during pregnancy to adjust their doses. Free drug levels are better guides than total serum levels.

FDA RISK CLASSIFICATION SYSTEM

Category A: Safety Established

Controlled studies in women do not show a risk to the fetus in the first trimester, there is no evidence of a risk in later trimesters, and the possibility of fetal harm appears remote.

Category B: Safety Likely

Either

Animal-reproduction studies have not demonstrated a foetal risk but there are no controlled studies in pregnant women. Or

Animal-reproduction studies have shown an adverse effect (other than a decrease in fertility) that was not confirmed in controlled studies in women in the first trimester and there is no evidence of a risk in later trimesters.

Category C: Teratogenicity Possible

Either Studies in animals have revealed adverse effects on the foetus (teratogenic, embryocidal, or other) and there are no controlled studies in women. Or

Studies in women and animals are not available. These drugs should be given only if the potential benefit justifies the potential risk to the foetus.

Category D: Teratogenicity Probable

There is positive evidence of human fetal risk, but the benefits from use in pregnant women may be acceptable despite the risk (e.g. if the drug is needed in a life-threatening situation or for a serious disease for which safer drugs cannot be used or are ineffective).

Category X: Teratogenicity likely—Contraindicated in Pregnancy

Studies in animals and humans have demonstrated fetal abnormalities and/or

There is evidence of fetal risk based on human experience and:

The risk of the use of the drug in pregnant women clearly outweighs any possible benefit. These drugs are contraindicated in women who are or may become pregnant.

Lactation

Breastfeeding has numerous health benefits for the baby. It

1. Optimizes nutrition
2. Limits exposure to foreign proteins
3. Provides necessary hormones, growth factors and immune complexes
4. Provides important fatty acids to facilitate good brain development
5. Reduces infant infections and mortality
6. Promotes maternal-baby bonding

Breastfeeding benefits to the nursing mother [7, 8, 9]

1. Assists with return to normal weight
2. Reduces risk for breast cancer
3. Reduces risk for ovarian cancer
4. Reduces risk for rheumatoid arthritis
5. Cost-effective method of supplying baby's nutrition
6. Improves maternal-baby bonding

Due to the numerous and substantial health benefits for both mother and baby from breastfeeding and the availability of relatively safe therapies, women should be encouraged to breastfeed and reassure mothers about the availability of safer, effective treatment options when nursing.

A variety of factors influence the likelihood that a maternal drug will affect the breastfed baby.

1. Timing of drug administration
2. Time to peak drug concentration
3. Drug half-life in both the mother and the baby
4. Drug bioavailability (the amount of medication that enters the blood)
5. Factors that influence how much drug appears in breast milk (e.g. molecular weight, as very large drugs are less likely to enter the breast milk)

There is wide range of variables in assessment of safety of drug during lactation.

1. Characteristics of the ingested drug, including medication pH and presence of active metabolites
2. Route of administration in the mother
3. Variability in maternal milk composition between and during feedings

SAFETY OF COMMONLY PRESCRIBED DRUGS IN PREGNANCY

NSAIDs in pregnancy[13]

Drug	FDA risk classification as per pregnancy trimester (1st/2nd/3rd)	Placental transfer	Indication
Acetaminophen	B/B/B	Yes	Fever, pain
Aspirin	D/D/D	Yes	Not recommended, except for specific conditions
Ibuprofen	B/B/D	Yes	Use with caution, avoid in 3rd trimester
Ketoprofen	B/B/D	Yes	Use with caution, avoid in 3rd trimester
Naproxen	B/B/D	Yes	Use with caution, avoid in 3rd trimester

Decongestants, expectorants and antihistamines in pregnancy[13]

Drug	FDA pregnancy risk classification	Drug class	Placental transfer	Indication
Chlorpheniramine	B	Antihistamine	Not known	Antihistamine of choice
Pseudoephedrine HCL	B	Decongestant	Not Known	Oral decongestant of choice, possible association with gastroschisis
Guaiphenisin	C	Expectorant	Not known	May be unsafe in first trimester
Dextromethorphan hydrobromide	C	Antitussive	Not known	Appears to be safe in pregnancy
Diphenhydramine	B	Antihistamine, antiemetic	Yes	Possible oxytocin-like effects at high dosages

Antidiarrhoeals in pregnancy[13]

Drug	FDA pregnancy risk classification	Placental transfer	Indication
Kaolin and pectin	B/B/B	No	Antidiarrheal of choice
Bismuth subsalicylate	C/C/D	Yes	Not recommended
Loperamide	B/B/B	Not known	Probably safe
Atropine/diphenoxylate	C/C/C	Not known	Not recommended

Antacids in pregnancy[13]

Drug	FDA pregnancy risk classification	Placental transfer	Indication
Aluminium hydroxide/magnesium hydroxide	B	Not known	Safe
Calcium carbonate	C	Not known	Safe
Cimetidine	B	Yes	Safe
Ranitidine	B	Yes	Safe
Famotidine	B	Yes	Probably safe

Topical vaginal antifungal in pregnancy[13]

Drug	FDA pregnancy risk classification	Placental transfer	Indication
Clotrimazole	C	Not known	Safe in 2nd and 3rd trimester, probably safe in 1st trimester
Miconazole	C	Not known	Probably safe

4. Variability in infant milk consumption and clearance

5. Most drugs enter the breast milk through passive diffusion, with transfer highest for fat-soluble drugs.

6. Milk is slightly more acidic than plasma, basic drugs are more likely to transfer into the breast milk.

7. Age of the baby.

These factors still do not help accurately estimating drug exposure. For example, the initial 10 ml of expressed milk during a feeding has about half of the fat content that will be seen with milk consumed later in the feeding.[10]

Consequently, a lower concentration of fat-soluble drugs will be present in the first milk of each feeding. In addition, glomerular filtration and drug metabolism are less robust in younger babies, resulting in lower drug clearance in babies until they are 6–12 months old.

Because of the wide range of patient and pharmacokinetic variables required to accurately measure a baby's true exposure, it is not feasible to calculate risk in most clinical settings individually. The milk-to-plasma ratio is a ratio of the level of drug in milk divided by the level of drug in maternal plasma.

Another method for quantifying the infant exposure through breast milk is the relative infant dose, which is calculated as a percentage of the infant dose to maternal dose.[11]

The relative infant dose is calculated by dividing the dose of the drug in milk (mg/kg/day) by the dose administered to the mother each day (mg/kg/day). In term infants, a relative infant dose <10% is generally considered to be safe with short-term use. A lower percentage is preferred for premature babies. In general, risk can be minimized by:

Safety of important medications in lactation[14]		
Drug	Effect on baby	Comments
Aspirin	Minimal	Occasional dose is safe, high dose is significant in milk
Ampicillin	Minimal	Possible occurrence of diarrhoea, allergic sensitization
Chloramphenicol	Significant	Gray baby syndrome at higher dosage with bone marrow suppression, hence not recommended
Chlorpromazine	Minimal	Insignificant quantity in breast milk
Diazepam	Significant	Causes sedation in infant
Digoxin	Minimal	Insignificant quantity in breast milk
Isoniazide	Minimal	Possibility of pyridoxine deficiency in infant
Lithium	Significant	Avoid breastfeeding
Oral contraceptives	Minimal	May suppress lactation at a high dose
Penicillin	Minimal	Very low concentration in milk
Phenobarbitone	Moderate	Hypnotic dose can cause sedation in infant
Phenytoin	Moderate	Concentration in breast milk is not sufficient to cause adverse effect
Prednisolone	Moderate	Low dose is safe. More than twice the physiologic dose should be avoided
Propranalol	Minimal	Very small amount in breast milk
Tetracycline	Moderate	Can cause permanent staining of teeth
Theophylline	Moderate	Not likely to produce significant effect
Tolbutamide	Minimal	Low concentration in breast milk
Warfarin	Minimal	Very small quantities in breast milk

1. Selecting drugs with poor transfer into breast milk (e.g. large molecular weight compounds)
2. Selecting drugs that are safe in babies
3. Timing maternal drug dosing to minimize exposure in the baby

Drugs that might affect the baby may still be used by the nursing mother if her doctor can identify how long a harmful concentration will be present in her milk following drug ingestion. In general, it is recommended that milk be pumped and dumped for approximately 4 half-lives of the ingested drug to reduce the concentration to safer levels for the baby.[12] For example, if the half-life of a drug is 2 hours, then the mother should pump and discard her milk for 8 hours after medication ingestion. The mother can then supplement the baby with either stored breast milk or formula during that time.

Also, when baby is sleeping through the night, mother can take her once daily medication immediately after baby's last feeding before bedtime and possibly dump her first supply of breast milk in the morning.

ANESTHESIA IN PREGNANCY

All the commonly used inhalational agents readily cross the placental barrier and the concentration in the fetal blood quickly approaches the levels in the mother. They also hinder uterine contraction and so increase the potential for postpartum hemorrhage. They are given in sub-anaesthetic concentration before the delivery of the baby and if hemorrhage secondary to uterine relaxation is present.

In general obstetric anesthesia involve the avoidance of agents or drugs that cross the placental barrier, depress fetal vital signs, cause myocardial or respiratory depression and initiate untimely uterine contractions.

REFERENCES

1. Koren G, Pastuszak A, Ito S. Drugs in pregnancy. *N Engl J Med.* 1998;338:1128–1137.
2. Collaborative Group on Drug Use in Pregnancy. An international survey on drug utilization during pregnancy. *Int J Risk Safety Med.* 1991;1:1.
3. Glover DD, Amonkar M, Rybeck BF, Tracy TS. Prescription, over-the-counter, and herbal medicine use in a rural, obstetric population. Am J Obstet Gynecol 2003;188:1039–1045.
4. Precht DH, Andersen PK, Olsen J. Severe life events and impaired fetal growth: A nationwide study with complete follow-up. Acta Obstet Gynecol Scand 2007;86:266–275.
5. Hansen D, Lou HC, Olsen J. Serious life events and congenital malformations: A national study with complete follow-up. Lancet 2000;356:875–880.
6. Scolnik D, Nulman I, Rovet J, et al. Neurodevelopment of children exposed in utero to phenytoin and carbamazepine monotherapy. *JAMA.* 1994;271:767–770.
7. Ip S, Chung M, Raman G, et al. Breastfeeding and maternal and infant health outcomesin developed countries. Evid Rep Technol Assess (Full Rep) 2007;135:1–186.
8. Pikwer M, Bergström U, Nilsson JA, et al. Breast-feeding, but not oral contraceptives, is associated with a reduced risk of rheumatoid arthritis. Ann Rheum Dis.
9. Sances G, Granella F, Nappi RE, et al. Course of migraine during pregnancy and postpartum: A prospective study. Cephalalgia 2003;23:197–205.
10. McNamara PJ, Abbassi M. Neonatal exposure to drugs in breast milk. Pharma Res 2004;21:555–566.
11. Lee KG. Lactation and drugs. Paediatrics Child Health 2007;17:68–71.
12. http://www.medsafe.govt.nz/Profs/PUarticles/lactation.html.
13. Ronald A. Black, MD, and D. Ashley HILL, MD Over-the-Counter Medications in Pregnancy American Family Physician, 2003; 67: 12: 2517–2526.
14. Koren G. Special aspects of Perinatal and paediatric pharmacology in Bertram G. Katzung, Basic and Clinical Pharmacology, 8th ed, 2000; 1025–1035.

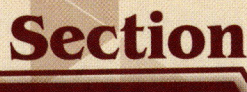

Section

II

Approach and Diagnostics

7

Clinical Clues: Fever with and without Rash

Parikshit D Tank

INTRODUCTION

The differential diagnosis of fever in pregnancy is broadly divided into conditions which are specifically related to pregnancy and those where the pregnant state is a coincidence. Though there are literally hundreds of possibilities, the etiology of fever in pregnancy can be narrowed down to a handful of common ones that are seen commonly in clinical practice. A smaller subgroup of women present with a rash (Table 7.1). This is an important clinical clue towards diagnosing the etiology. A fever with rash in pregnancy should alert the clinician of the specific infections that could have fetal implications. This chapter is limited to the clinical aspects of evaluating women with fever in pregnancy.

CLINICAL APPROACH

The clinical clues and the approach to the pregnant woman should be directed towards:

Table 7.1: Common etiologies and clinical approach to fever in pregnancy				
Fever with obstetric	*Fever with site*	*Fever with systemic*	*Fever in typical*	*Fever with rash*
Features (amniotic fluid leak, long-standing fetal death, uterine pain or tenderness) present	Specific features predominating the clinical picture	Features predominating, general condition is affected	Patterns (not commonly seen when treatments are initiated early, antipyretics are used)	
Chorioamnionitis	Respiratory infections	Viral fever	Malaria—tertian or quotidian	Measles
Puerperal sepsis	Urinary infections	Malaria	TB—evening rise of temperature	Rubella
	Gastroenteritis	Dengue	Typhoid—step ladder pattern	Chickenpox
	Mastitis or breast abscess	Hepatitis	Puerperal sepsis, iliac vein thrombo-phlebitis—hectic temperature patterns	Herpes simplex
	Meningitis or cerebral malaria Hepatitis	Leptospirosis		Parvovirus

- Assessing maternal condition and stability
- Ascertaining fetal viability and well-being
- Directing investigations based on the clinical picture

Assessing Maternal Condition and Stability

A primary goal in caring for women presenting with fever is to assess their general condition and stability. It guides the clinician on the following aspects:

- Is there a recordable fever? This is an important question that should be answered in women who have only a sensation of warmth and are otherwise healthy. Pregnancy, with the raised basal metabolic rate induces such a sensation of warmth. There is often fatigue and lassitude accompanying it. An objectively recorded fever should be present before pursuing.
- A detailed history focusing on the progress of symptoms, pattern of fever and systemic features is an invaluable tool. The pattern of fever is typical in certain etiologies

described (Table 7.2). However, these typical patterns may not always hold good when antipyretic and antibiotic use is initiated before presentation to the doctor.

- Need for inpatient admission and intensive care—based on general condition and vital parameters, possible diagnosis or as dictated by investigations. Women with features outlined (Table 7.3) should be offered admission.
- Need for a consultation with a physician, surgeon or other specialist depending on the general condition, vital parameters and site specific features.
- Signs in the general examination (icterus, increased respiratory rate, skin rashes).
- To look for site specific symptoms and systemic examination.

Systemic examination should, at the bare minimum, look for the following:

- Neurological—headaches, altered sensorium, altered behavior, convulsions on history. Examination may reveal meningism, neck rigidity and signs of increased intracranial pressure.

Table 7.2: Fever patterns and etiology

Pattern	Description	Typical etiology
Quotidian, tertian, quartan	Fever occurring daily, every other day or every third day respectively in paroxysms	Malaria
Evening rise of temperature	Low grade fever of about 100 degrees F occurring in the evening	Tuberculosis
Step ladder pattern	Rising temperatures with new peaks and not returning to baseline	Typhoid
Hectic	Very high temperatures (>104 degrees F) with normal recordings in irregular spikes	Bacteremia from a specific focus such as an abscess, thrombophlebitis

Table 7.3: Indications for admission for women with fever in pregnancy

Temperature	> 102 degrees F
Vital parameters	Pulse < 60 or > 120 bpm, respirations <14 or >22 /min, hypotension or hypertension, SpO_2 < 95%
Systemic features	Neurological—convulsions, altered consciousness, focal features, jaundice, severe abdominal pain, dehydration, oliguria
Social	Poor access to investigations or follow up, compliance is in doubt, not responding to primary line of treatment

- Respiratory—running nose, cough, pain in the throat, sinuses and ears should be sought on history. Look for wheezing, unequal air entry and rales on examination.
- Abdomen—vomiting, diarrhea, pain and spasms are usually common features. An enlarged spleen and/or liver in early pregnancy might give diagnostic clues to malaria or hepatitis. Site specific tenderness (right upper abdomen—cholecystitis, McBurney's point—appendicitis, loin to groin pain—pyelonephritis) should be looked for, but due to the enlarging uterus, location may not be specific.
- Urinary—Urgency and incontinence are often seen in pregnancy without urinary infection. However, pain and burning during urination are generally indicative of an infection.
- In a postpartum woman with fever, breast examination should be done to rule out mastitis or a breast abscess.

FEVER WITH RASH

Pregnant women who present with fever and rash are a special subset. A complete clinical evaluation can be useful in identify the offending agent. Details regarding possible sources of exposure such as an index case with similar features in the household or workplace should be obtained. The chronology of events in terms of exposure, onset of fever, rash and other symptoms should be established. On examination, one should look for typical patterns of rash and involvement of other systems. A simplified table is presented for quick reference (Table 7.4). The differential diagnosis and some leading features of a patient presenting with fever and rash are:

Typical Presentations

1. Measles—upper respiratory complaints, conjunctivitis, Koplik spots on buccal mucosa, maculopapular rash first on the face and neck and then on the trunk.
2. Rubella (German measles)—catarrh, transient macular rash on the face spreading to the trunk, non-tender posterior cervical, auricular and suboccipital lymphadenopathy.
3. Varicella zoster (Chickenpox)— progressive centrifugal rash with macules, papules, vesicles, pustules and scabs occurring together.
4. Herpes simplex—painful blisters in dermatomal distribution in orofacial (HSV1) or genital (HSV2) regions.
5. Syphilis—Secondary syphilis causes roseolar rash with grayish white moist mucus patches in the oropharynx.
6. Parvovirus B19—fine reticular rash involving the face (slapped cheeks appearance), arthralgia.
   - *Atypical presentations:* Malaria, miliary tuberculosis, hepatitis A, drug rash, HIV associated skin lesions, Staphylococcus

Table 7.4: Fever with rash—a quick reference		
Pregnancy rash	*Non-specific rash of viral fevers*	*Specific patterns*
Usually late pregnancy	Widespread	Chickenpox–starts on the trunk (centrifugal), varied morphology
Itching	Transient	
Flat papules	Macules	
Non-specific location		
		Measles—starts on the face (centripetal), maculo-pappular
		Herpes simplex—specific locations (labial, genital), painful, vesicular
		Parvovirus B19—slapped cheek rash (not easily identifiable in dark skinned), arthralgia

induced toxic shock syndrome (TSS), Typhoid.

- *Rare diseases:* Lyme disease, murine typhus, Q fever, coxsackie B virus, echovirus, leptospirosis.

FETAL VIABILITY AND WELL-BEING

Even as the maternal evaluation and care should be primary, an assessment of the fetus should be done as per the gestational age. This might include assessing the uterine size, auscultation of the fetal heart beat, electronic fetal monitoring or using ultrasound for confirming viability, liquor and biophysical profile. In most conditions, the fetal status is not affected and fetal assessment is secondary. However, it is an important consideration for the mother and a reassuring status would put her at ease.

CLINICAL ASPECTS OF COMMON INVESTIGATIONS

In otherwise well patients where the clinical diagnosis is obviously a mild upper respiratory tract infection or a viral fever, there may not be a role for conducting any investigation. The common investigations are discussed in another chapter. Some clinical aspects of the tests that are relevant are mentioned below:

- Complete blood count should almost always be done
- Ideally, blood for peripheral smear for malaria should be drawn when the fever is present. However, this may not always be possible if the patient is not admitted. In this situation, it may be useful to request two samples 12 hours apart.

- Urine routine and microscopy—a first urine sample in the morning gives better diagnostic yield. Urine should be collected after cleaning the vulva with soap and water. A midstream urine sample should be collected.
- X-ray chest with an abdominal shield can safely be performed even in the first trimester of pregnancy if the clinical situation demands it. The information and benefit to be gained by a positive diagnosis of tuberculosis and its subsequent treatment far outweigh any theoretical concerns of harming the fetus.
- If neurological imaging is essential, MRI should be preferred over a CT scan. Ionizing contrast material should be avoided.

BIBLIOGRAPHY

1. Stirrat G. The immune system. In: Clinical Physiology in Obstetrics. Eds: Hytten F, Chamberlain G. London, Blackwell, 1991; p 101.
2. Towbin JA. Presentation and diagnosis of fetal infection. In: High Risk Pregnancy Management Options 2nd edn. Eds: James DK, Steer PJ, Weiner CP, Gonik B. London, Harcourt Publishers Limited 1999; pp 519–524.
3. Salvi VS, Tank PD. Infections and Vaccines in the First Trimester—Issues in Management. In: Medical and Surgical Disorders in Pregnancy. Ed: Salvi VS. New Delhi, FOGSI Jaypee Brothers, 2003, pp 178–186.
4. Tank PD. Other Infections in Pregnancy. In: Medical and Surgical Disorders in Pregnancy. Ed: Salvi VS. New Delhi, FOGSI Jaypee Brothers, 2003, pp 202–206.
5. Vakil RJ, Golwalla AF. Physical diagnosis: A textbook of symptoms and physical signs. 15th ed. MPP, Mumbai; 2014.

8

Approach to Viral Fever
(Physicians Perspective)

Om Shrivastav

BACKGROUND

Viral infections in pregnancy are major causes of maternal and fetal morbidity and mortality. Infections can develop in the neonate transplacentally, perinatally (from vaginal secretions or blood), or postnatally (from breast milk or other sources).

Infections known to produce congenital defects have been described with the acronym TORCH [*Toxoplasma*, others, rubella, cytomegalovirus (CMV), herpes].

Traditionally, the only viral infections of concern during pregnancy were those caused by rubella virus, CMV, and herpes simplex virus (HSV). Other viruses now known to cause congenital infections include parvovirus B19 (B19V), varicella-zoster virus (VZV), West Nile virus, measles virus, enteroviruses, adenovirus, and human immunodeficiency virus (HIV).

Also of importance is hepatitis E virus because of the high mortality rate associated with infection in pregnant women. Recently, lymphocytic choriomeningitis virus (LCMV) has been implicated as a teratogenic rodent-borne arenavirus.

CYTOMEGALOVIRUS

Geographic location, socioeconomic class, and work exposure are other factors that influence the risk of infection. CMV infection requires intimate contact through saliva, urine, and/or other body fluids. Possible routes of transmission include sexual contact, organ transplantation, transplacental transmission, transmission via breast milk, and blood transfusion.

Primary, reactivation, or recurrent CMV infection can occur in pregnancy and can lead to congenital CMV infection. Transplacental infection can result in intrauterine growth restriction, and several CNS and ENT manifestations including:

- Sensorineural hearing loss
- Intracranial calcifications
- Microcephaly, hydrocephalus
- Hepatosplenomegaly
- Delayed psychomotor development, and/or optic atrophy.

First trimester infections are the severest, though vertical transmission of CMV can occur at any stage of pregnancy; while the overall risk of infection is greatest in the third trimester. The risk of transmission to the fetus in primary infection is 30–40%. Most (90%) CMV infections cause no symptoms.

Thirty percent of infants will succumb to severe CMV. Congenital hearing loss is the most common sequel of recurrent CMV infection.

HERPES SIMPLEX VIRUS

One-third to half of women receiving obstetric care have serologic evidence of past HSV infection. Although both HSV-1 and HSV-2 may cause neonatal herpes, HSV-2 is responsible for 70% of cases. Neonatal herpetic infection is defined as infection within 28 days of birth. Ninety percent of infections are perinatally transmitted in the birth canal. HSV infection acquired in this manner is associated with 3 distinct syndromes, each with its own typical outcome.

The first and most common (45%) is localized skin, eye, or mouth disease.

Approximately 30% of cases manifest as central nervous system (CNS) disease, including meningitis or encephalitis, with evidence of HSV DNA in the cerebrospinal fluid (CSF).

Finally, 25% of neonatal herpetic infections manifest as disseminated disease that involves multiple organs. Initial symptoms of this disease usually present during the first 4 weeks of life.

Approximately 10% of infections are congenital, usually a consequence of the mother acquiring primary HSV infection during pregnancy.

The risk of neonatal herpes and death is highest in infants born to mothers who have not seroconverted by the time of delivery.

RUBELLA

Congenital rubella syndrome (CRS) is characterized by:

- Intrauterine growth restriction
- Intracranial calcifications
- Microcephaly
- Cataracts
- Cardiac defects (most commonly patent ductus arteriosus or pulmonary arterial hypoplasia)
- Neurologic disease (with a broad range of presentations, from behavior disorders to meningoencephalitis)
- Osteitis, and
- Hepatosplenomegaly.

Neonates with rubella may have a "blueberry muffin" appearance caused by purpuric skin lesions that result from extramedullary hematopoiesis.

Heart defects in these infants include ventricular septal defects, patent ductus arteriosus, pulmonary stenosis, and coarctation of the aorta. Complications develop in infants born to mothers who acquire rubella infection during the first 16 weeks of pregnancy. Ninety percent of infants present with some finding of congenital rubella if infection occurs within the first 12 weeks, and 20% present with congenital disease if the infection occurs between weeks 12 and 16.

PARVOVIRUS B19

B19 infections in fetus have profound effects on both, and the clinical syndrome is called erythema infectiosum (fifth disease). Although most adults with B19V infection are asymptomatic, the effects of this virus on the fetus are much greater and include:

- Miscarriage
- Fetal anemia
- Hydrops fetalis
- Myocarditis and/or
- Intrauterine fetal death
- B19V infection accounts for 15–20% of cases of nonimmune hydrops fetalis.

VARICELLA-ZOSTER VIRUS

VZV is a common virus that carries risks for both the mother and fetus during pregnancy. Morbidity and mortality rates associated with VZV infection are much higher in adults than in children.

Primary varicella infection during pregnancy is considered a medical emergency. Pneumonitis due to VZV infection is 25 times more common in adults than in children. Other risk factors for the development of pneumonitis include:
- Smoking and
- A large lesion burden (>100 lesions).

Congenital varicella syndrome (CVS) results in spontaneous abortion, chorioretinitis, cataracts, limb atrophy, cerebral cortical atrophy, and/or neurological disability. Spontaneous abortion has been reported in 3–8% of first-trimester VZV infections.

ENTEROVIRUS

Enterovirus infections are not believed to cross the placenta and cause fetal disease. However, some studies have linked coxsackie virus and echovirus to miscarriage, neuro-developmental delay, myocarditis, and cortical necrosis. One study linked the presence of coxsackievirus in the third trimester with respiratory failure and global cognitive defects.

MEASLES VIRUS

Measles virus infection (rubeola) during pregnancy has a pneumonitis predominating presentation. Although it is not known to be teratogenic, rubeola has been associated with spontaneous abortion, premature labor, and low birth weight.

LYMPHOCYTIC CHORIOMENINGITIS VIRUS

LCMV has been associated with sporadic cases of congenital infection worldwide. Affected infants demonstrate chorioretinitis, hydrocephalus, mental retardation, and/or visual impairment; in addition, intrauterine death is possible. Unlike congenital CMV and rubella infections, hearing deficits and hepatosplenomegaly are rarely seen in congenital LCMV.

OTHER VIRUSES

Other viruses postulated to cause congenital infections include:
- Echovirus
- Hepatitis B virus
- Hepatitis C virus, and
- Adenovirus.
- Clinical presentation

The hallmark of diagnosis of congenital disease is maternal history and history of any recent exposures to ill individuals, physical findings in the newborn, and appropriate laboratory testing. The maternal immunization history is also extremely important.

WORKUP

Laboratory Studies

Careful interpretation of serologic markers for most of these infections is important. Immunoglobulin M (IgM) can persist for up to a year, leading to difficulty in determining fetal exposure during pregnancy.

Serology for CMV can be difficult to interpret. Although 50–80% of women may have serological findings of a past infection, this is not completely protective against reinfection.

A 4-fold or greater rise in the CMV-IgG titer within 2 weeks is consistent with a recent infection.

Assessing for avidity of the IgG antibody has also been useful to differentiate primary and recurrent CMV infection. Low-to-moderate avidity IgG antibody is more likely to represent an acute infection. CMV infection is best diagnosed with urine culture or polymerase chain reaction (PCR) using urine or serum. Rapid virus isolation in cell cultures (shell vial) is also highly sensitive and specific.

Amniocentesis for CMV PCR; after 21 weeks gestation; testing fetal serum for IgM antibodies is highly sensitive for congenital infection. identification of CMV in the amniotic fluid by culture or CMV is the most sensitive and specific test for congenital CMV.

Type-specific antibodies to HSV-1 and HSV-2 are used to confirm past exposure and current infection in the mother.

The most sensitive test for detecting HSV is cell culture, which is used to isolate the virus in tissue. PCR can be used to diagnose lesions found during pregnancy.

Papanicolaou tests and Tzanck tests are poor HSV-screening tests.

HSV PCR of amniotic fluid is sensitive but may not correlate with neonatal HSV infection.

In newborns with suspected disease, cultures of the skin lesions, mouth, eyes, urine, blood, stool, rectum, and CSF should be obtained. PCR can be used to detect HSV in the spinal fluid.

Traditionally, B19V infection has been confirmed with serological testing.

IgM may be present 10–12 days after exposure and can persist for up to 6 months, while IgG antibodies are formed by 3 weeks and may persist for years, primary varicella confers lifelong immunity. However, the diagnosis is usually made clinically. IgM can appear as soon as 3 days after the onset of symptoms.

Viral culture can be performed using skin lesions, or PCR for VZV DNA can be performed using specimens. There is poor correlation with fetal sequelae from VZV infection.

Diagnosis of VZV infection in the infant is difficult because only 27% have an IgM response.

Rubella—serum IgM levels peak 7–10 days after the onset of clinical illness and can persist for 6 weeks before declining. IgG can be detected within 2–3 weeks of infection.

Cordocentesis is difficult before 20 weeks gestation, and fetal immunoglobulins usually go undetected before 22 weeks gestation.

Although these tests can reveal rubella virus in the fetus, they do not indicate the degree of fetal injury.

Coxsackievirus infection can be confirmed by serology in the mother. *In situ* hybridization or reverse-transcriptase PCR of tissue can be performed on the newborn, measles virus infection can be confirmed by IgM serology.

LCMV infection can be diagnosed based on an IgM enzyme-linked immunosorbent assay (ELISA) of CSF or serum. CSF pressure is generally increased, with protein levels of 50–300 mg/dL and lymphocytes. Patients may also exhibit leukopenia or thrombocytopenia.

Diagnosis of influenza in pregnancy should be based on clinical symptoms without waiting for diagnostic tests

Imaging

Fetal ultrasonography can be used to diagnose growth restriction and may reveal specific findings.

If a mother tests positive for B19V IgM and negative for IgG, suggesting a new infection, she should undergo serial ultrasonography to monitor for development of fetal anemia for 10–12 weeks after exposure. Fetal demise is most likely if infection occurs before 20 weeks' gestation.

Doppler assessment shows elevated middle cerebral artery peak systolic velocity (MCA-PSV) in cases of fetal anemia.

Elevated MCA-PSV values warrant fetal blood sampling to assess the degree of anemia and intrauterine transfusion, if necessary.

Chest radiography—diffuse peribronchial nodular infiltrates and interstitial pneumonitis.

Prenatal diagnosis of varicella 5 or more weeks following the initial time of suspected VZV infection in the first trimester.

- Hypoplasia
- Stippling of the epiphyseal plates
- Club-foot deformities
- Ventriculomegaly
- Patent ductus arteriosus

DIAGNOSTIC PROCEDURES

Amniocentesis or chorionic villous sampling can assist in confirming infections with rubella virus, CMV, B19V, and possibly, HSV.

GENITAL HERPES IN PREGNANCY

Genital HSV Infections

HSV is a DNA virus. HSV has 2 subtypes: Herpes simplex virus 1 (HSV-1) and HSV-2. Although each is a distinct virus, they share some antigenic components, such that antibodies that react to one type may "neutralize" the other.

HSV-1 infections were traditionally associated with the oral area (fever blisters), whereas HSV-2 infections occurred in the genital region. Currently, approximately 15% of genital HSV infections are caused by HSV-1.

The following 4 designations are given for genital HSV infections:

- Primary
- Nonprimary first-episode
- Recurrent
- Asymptomatic viral shedding

Primary Infections

Typically, lesions appear 2–14 days after exposure. Without antiviral therapy, the lesions usually last for 20 days.

Antibody response occurs 3–4 weeks after the infection and is lifelong. However, unlike protective antibodies to other viruses, antibodies to HSV do not prevent local recurrence.

The lesions of a primary infection begin as tender vesicles, which may rupture and become ulcers. The vaginal mucosa is commonly inflamed and edematous. The cervix is involved in 70–90% of patients.

Symptoms associated with primary infections may be both local and constitutional. Local symptoms include intense pain, dysuria, itching, vaginal discharge, and lymphadenopathy. Constitutional symptoms are due to viremia and include fever, headache, nausea, malaise, and myalgia.

Importantly, more than 75% of patients with primary genital HSV infection are asymptomatic.

Nonprimary First-episode Infections

A nonprimary first-episode infection is a first genital HSV outbreak in a woman who has heterologous HSV antibodies. The duration of lesions is also shorter (averaging 15 days),

and shedding lasts for only approximately 7 days.

Distinguishing primary infections from nonprimary first-episode infections by clinical presentation is difficult. Instead, the diagnosis is based on type-specific culture and type-specific serology. The absence of any HSV antibodies at the time of the outbreak confirms a primary infection, whereas antibody to the heterologous HSV type confirms a nonprimary first-episode infection.

Recurrent Infections

Approximately 15% of all pregnant women with a history of genital HSV infection experience recurrent lesions at delivery. Recurrent HSV outbreaks may be symptomatic or asymptomatic. When present, most symptoms are localized (e.g. pain, itching, vaginal discharge).

Lesions typically last for 9 days, and shedding lasts for approximately 4 days. Shedding is usually completed before the lesions resolve.

ASYMPTOMATIC VIRAL SHEDDING

Asymptomatic viral shedding is episodic and brief, usually lasting 24-48 hours. One to 2% of pregnant women with a history of recurrent HSV infection have asymptomatic shedding at the time of delivery. Coinfection with HIV may increase asymptomatic shedding of HSV in women.

PERINATAL TRANSMISSION OF HSV

HSV can be vertically transmitted to the infant before, during, or after delivery, although intrapartum transmission accounts for most cases. Maternal age of less than 21 years is a risk factor for vertical transmission.[6]

ANTENATAL

Approximately 5% of all cases of neonatal HSV infection result from in utero transmission.

Hematogenous spread can produce a spectrum of findings similar to other TORCH (toxoplasmosis, other infections, rubella, cytomegalovirus, and herpes simplex) infections, such as microcephaly, microphthalmia, intracranial calcifications, and chorioretinitis.

INTRAPARTUM

Intrapartum transmission accounts for most neonatal infections and occurs with passage of the infant through an infected birth canal. The use of a fetal-scalp electrode increases the risk for intrapartum transmission. From 75% to 90% of infants with neonatal HSV are born to infected asymptomatic mothers who have no known history of genital HSV.

POSTNATAL

Postnatal transmission of HSV can occur through contact with infected parents or healthcare workers.

PERINATAL TRANSMISSION RATES

Viral shedding in labor.
- Neonatal transmission is highest in women who are seronegative, confirming the importance of maternal antibodies in preventing neonatal transmission.

- The presence of HSV-2 antibodies appears to reduce not only neonatal HSV-2 infections (no neonatal HSV infections from 140 recurrent shedders) but also maternal HSV-1 infections (i.e. no cases of non-primary HSV-1 infections).
- Rates of neonatal HSV infection, both primary and recurrent, are greater with HSV-1 than with HSV-2.
- Cesarean delivery is protective against neonatal infection, confirming a long-standing practice that had never previously been scientifically validated.

HSV DETECTION METHODS

HSV Culture

Sensitivity of 70% and a specificity of nearly 100%. The culture yield is highest during the prodrome and lowest during the second half of the outbreak, especially with recurrent lesions.

Tzank Smear

The Tzank smear is now of historical interest only.

Polymerase Chain Reaction

Like the viral culture, PCR can distinguish HSV-1 from HSV-2. The test takes approximately

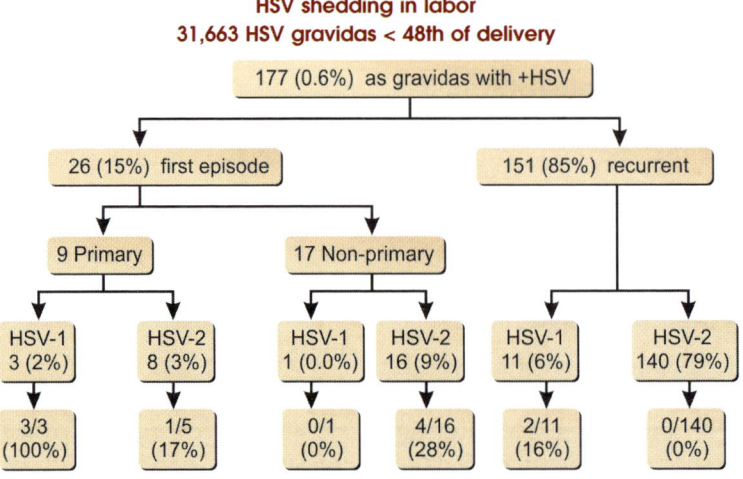

1 day for results to be returned and has the potential for a higher detection rate than HSV culture.

PCR does not differentiate actively replicating HSV from latent HSV DNA.

ANTIVIRAL THERAPY

Acyclovir

Acyclovir is selective for HSV-infected cells because it requires phosphorylation by a viral enzyme (thymidine kinase) to acyclovir monophosphate. Phosphorylation does not occur in uninfected cells, where it remains virtually undetectable.

With primary HSV infection in nonpregnant women, acyclovir reduces the duration of local pain, dysuria, and viral shedding, and it shortens the time to crusting and healing of lesions. With daily usage, acyclovir also reduces symptomatic recurrences and subclinical viral shedding.

During pregnancy, acyclovir crosses the placenta and concentrates in the amniotic fluid. Postpartum, acyclovir concentrates in breast milk. Fetal serum concentrations are equivalent to maternal serum concentrations.

Valacyclovir and Famciclovir

Both valacyclovir and famciclovir have been labeled category B drugs.

The recommended dosages of the 3 antiviral agents are given in Table 8.1.

Historical approach: Weekly cervical cultures of asymptomatic women with history of genital HSV.

The Infectious Disease Society for Obstetrics and Gynecology developed a position statement that recommended the following practices:

- Abandon weekly cervical cultures.
- In the absence of active lesions or prodromal symptoms, vaginal delivery should be allowed.
- At the time of delivery, consider obtaining a herpes culture from the mother or the neonate for the benefit of the pediatricians.
- Herpes cultures, when obtained, should be obtained from the cervix and the site of recurrence.
- If there is an active herpetic lesion, cesarean delivery should be performed, preferably within 4–6 hours of membrane rupture.
- If there is a recent infection near term, check cervical cultures every 3–5 days until results are negative.

Current Strategies to Prevent Vertical HSV Transmission

Current strategies to prevent vertical transmission with antiviral therapy have focused on 3 approaches, as follows:

- Antiviral suppression for gravidas with first-episode infections during pregnancy
- Routine antiviral suppression for gravidas with a history of genital HSV
- Identification of seronegative gravidas at risk for primary and nonprimary first-episode genital HSV infections

Antiviral suppression for gravidas with first-episode infections during pregnancy.

Routine antiviral suppression for gravidas with a history of genital HSV.

All of the observed outcomes were significantly reduced with suppressive use of acyclovir (no 95% confidence interval included the value of 1). No cases of neonatal herpes were reported in any of the 799 infants in all 5 studies, whether in the acyclovir or

Indication	Acyclovir	Valacyclovir	Famciclovir
First episode	400 mg tid *or* 200 mg 5 times/d (for 7–10 d)	1000 mg bid (for 7–10 d)	250 mg tid (for 7–10 d)
Recurrent	400 mg tid (for 3–5 d) *or* 800 mg PO tid (for 2 d)	500 mg bid (for 3 d)	1000 mg bid (for 1 d)

Table 8.1: Recommended dosages of the antiviral agents for genital herpes infection

Table 8.2: Antiviral trial results

Outcome	Acyclovir, %	Placebo, %	OR (95% CI)
Recurrent HSV infection at delivery	3.5	15.5	.25 (.15–.40)
Cesarean deliveries for HSV	4.0	14.7	.30 (.13–.67)
Total cesarean deliveries	16.7	25.9	.61 (.43–.86)
Asymptomatic HSV shedding at delivery	0	3.1	.09 (.02–.39)

placebo group (Table 8.2). Due to the rarity of neonatal HSV infections, far larger numbers of subjects are required to demonstrate a significant difference in this important outcome.

Identification of Seronegative Gravidas at risk for Primary and Nonprimary First-episode Genital HSV Infections

If routine serologic screening revealed that a woman was at risk for primary HSV (no antibodies) or nonprimary first-episode infection (either HSV-1 or HSV-2 only), she could be counseled to avoid genital-genital or oral-genital contact in order to prevent new genital infections during the third trimester of pregnancy and, hence, reduce neonatal HSV infections.

An alternative strategy would be to check the serologic status of the sexual partner, as well, and to recommend sexual abstinence only if the woman was at risk and the couple was serologically discordant, which occurs in 15–25% of couples. For example, if a woman was seronegative for HSV-2, and her partner was seropositive for HSV-2, the woman's risk of acquiring HSV-2 during pregnancy would be as high as 20%. Such a couple would, thus, be advised to abstain from sexual activity during pregnancy.

9

Diagnostic Modalities— An Update

Sandhya Sawant, Jayanthi Shastri

INTRODUCTION

Fever in pregnancy refers to an elevated temperature, often associated with other symptoms. In pregnant women, most infections are no more serious than in non-pregnant women of similar age. Infections during pregnancy affect the mother and often the child, either in utero or at the time of delivery. Many infections have been linked with increased risk of premature delivery and low birth weight and associated morbidity and mortality. Infectious illnesses and fevers in the mother must be treated as any other serious illness.

The effect of fever on pregnancy depends upon the extent of temperature elevation, its duration, and the stage of fetal development when it occurs. Mild exposures during the pre-implantation period and more severe exposures during embryonic and fetal development often result in miscarriage, premature labor, growth restriction and stillbirth. Infections in pregnancy may be viral, bacterial or protozoan, affecting both mother and fetus.

The causes of fever in pregnancy, including both infectious and non-infectious, are as follows:

a. Bacterial and Opportunistic Infections

1. Gonococcal
   - Septicaemia
   - Salpingitis
   - Arthritis
2. Secondary syphilis
3. Gas gangarene
4. Tetanus
5. Opportunistic—associated with immune deficiency syndrome:
   - Candidiosis
   - Cryptococcosis
   - Histoplasmosis
   - Aspergillosis
   - Coccidioidomycosis

b. Systemic Diseases

1. Tuberculosis
2. Gall bladder
   - Cholecystitis
   - Cholangitis
   - Empyema
3. Abscesses
   - Dental
   - Breast
   - Subphrenic
   - Hepatic
   - Pelvic
   - Cerebral
4. Gastrointestinal
   - Appendicitis
   - Diverticulitis
5. Urinary tract infections
6. Retroperitoneal infection

7. Septicemia
   - Meningococcal
   - Streptococcal
   - Staphylococcal
   - Gonococcal
   - Listeriosis
   - Vibriosis
   - Brucellosis
8. Endocarditis
9. Breast
   - Mastitis
10. Other
   - Q-fever
   - Amebiasis
   - Leptospirosis
   - Dengue
   - Malaria

c. Non-infectious Causes

1. Neoplasms
   - Lymphoma
   - Leukemia
   - Melanoma
   - Metastasis
   - Retroperitoneal sarcoma
   - Tumors of the lung, kidney, pancreas, liver
2. Connective tissue disease
   - Rheumatic fever
   - Systemic lupus erythematosis
   - Rheumatoid arthritis
3. Other
   - Drug fever
   - Thromboembolism
   - Sarcoidosis
   - Hemolytic disease

This chapter is used to describe these infections, their modes of transmission, and their maternal and fetal effects (Table 9.1).

CLINICAL PRESENTATIONS

In general, perinatal infections have more severe fetal consequences when they occur early in gestation, because first-trimester infections may disrupt organogenesis. Second- and third-trimester infections can cause neurologic impairment or growth disturbances. In utero infection may be associated with certain ultrasound findings, such as intrauterine growth restriction, echogenic bowel, intracranial or intrahepatic calcifications, hydrocephalus, microcephaly, isolated ascites, pericardial or pleural effusions, or nonimmune hydrops, although congenital infections may be asymptomatic, and difficult to detect on ultrasound.

INTRA-AMNIOTIC INFECTION

Intra-amniotic (chorioamnionitis) infection of the chorion, amnion, amniotic fluid, placenta, or a combination. Infection increases risk of obstetric complications and problems in the fetus and neonate. Symptoms include fever, uterine tenderness, foul-smelling vaginal discharge, and maternal and fetal tachycardia.

Microorganisms, such as group B Streptococcus, *Listeria monocytogenes*, are implicated more frequently in intra-amniotic infection. Other organisms that have been reported in association with intra-amniotic infection include *Ureaplasma urealyticum*, Candida species; the most common high virulence isolates are Bacteroides species, and *Escherichia coli*.

Consider analyzing and culturing amniotic fluid if women have refractory preterm labor or preterm PROM. Treat intra-amniotic infections with broad spectrum antibiotics plus delivery.

URINARY TRACT INFECTIONS

Urinary tract infections (UTIs) are common during pregnancy. About 5–7% of women have been reported to have urinary infection without any symptoms. Such symptomatic bacteruria undetected and untreated may lead to symptomatic infection later in pregnancy, pyelonephritis and hypertension in pregnant woman as well as prematurity and perinatal death of fetus. The organisms that cause UTIs

Table 9.1: Causative agents, mode of transmission, and effects on mother and fetus/neonate

Causative agent	Mode of transmission	Effect on mother	Effect on fetus/newborn bacterial
Treponema pallidum	Intrauterine	Primary (asymptomatic, chancre, lymphadenopathy), secondary (rash, condylomata, alopecia, arthritis, periostitis, optic neuritis, interstitial keratitis, iritis, uveitis, meningitis) and tertiary (cardiovascular, neurological, joint disorders, gummas, dementia)	Abortion, stillbirth, premature birth followed by live births of infants with stigmata of syphilis and finally healthy infant.
Listeria monocytogenes	Mostly intrauterine, perinatal. Soil, food, animals	Headache, myalgia, fever, loin pains, pharyngitis, gastro-intestinal symptoms	Fetal death, chronic intra-uterine, congenital or peri-natal infection, prematurity, meningoencephalitis
Mycobacterium tuberculosis	Mostly intrauterine, postnatal	Low grade fever, malaise, night sweats, weight loss, usually respiratory symptoms	Abortion, premature birth, stillbirth
Viral			
Coxsackie A and B	Mostly intrauterine	Herpangina; hand, foot, mouth disease; myocardiopathy, aseptic meningitis, Bornholm disease	Abortion, stillbirth, neonatal sepsis, myocarditis-meningo-encephalitis
Cytomegalovirus	Mostly intrauterine and through breast milk	Usually asymptomatic. Some-times moderate to high fever in primary infection	Deafness, microcephaly, hepatosplenomegaly, jaundice, hydrops fetalis
Echovirus		Rash may resemble rubella; mimics appendicitis and abruption placenta	Neonatal sepsis, disseminated infection (hepatic necrosis), late stillbirth
Hepatitis B	Intrauterine, post-natal, mostly perinatal. HBsAg positive mother (60–90%)	HBsAg positive mother (5–15 %)	Do not suffer from any clinical illness but remain carriers for life
Hepatitis C	Intrauterine, mostly perinatal, depends on HCV RNA-titres.		No apparent clinical illness
Herpes simplex	Intrauterine and perinatal. Postnatal in HSV 1	Oral or genital papular eruptions; more severe in pregnancy	Abortion after primary infection, fatal disseminated infection, prematurity, congenital malformations, stillbirth, intrauterine growth restriction
Human Immunodefi-ciency viruses (HIV-1&2)	Intrauterine, postnatal, mostly perinatal	Asymptomatic, unless had AIDS	Recurrent bacterial infections, failure to thrive, chronic diarrhea, lymphadenopathy

Contd...

Causative agent	Mode of transmission	Effect on mother	Effect on fetus/newborn bacterial
Table 9.1: Causative agents, mode of transmission, and effects on mother and fetus/neonate (*Contd...*)			
Influenza	Intrauterine and postnatal	Up to 54% mortality in pandemics	Uncertain.
Measles	Mostly intrauterine	May be complicated by pneumonia and CCF. More severe. May be fatal	Congenital measles, increased mortality
Mumps	Intrauterine	Nonspecific effects	Increased mortality, endocardial fibroelastosis
Rubella (German measles)	Mostly intrauterine, postnatal	Mild nonspecific symptoms	Congenital malformations, abortions, fetal death, chronic infection
Parvovirus B19	Intrauterine	Asymptomatic "slapped-cheek" rash, erythema infectiosum (fifth disease)	Second trimester abortions, hydrops fetalis due to severe anemia, myocarditis, hepatitis, hematological effects in late pregnancy
Varicella zoster (Chickenpox)	Intrauterine and perinatal	More severe; maternal death	Varicella embryopathy, congenital 1 varicella syndrome, infantile zoster, microcephaly focal brain calcification, optic atrophy, skin scarring, limb atrophy
Protozoal			
Plasmodium species	Intrauterine	Increased susceptibility. Maternal death, anemia	Abortion, stillbirth, premature delivery, intrauterine growth restriction, low birth weight.
Toxoplasma gondii	Intrauterine	Usually asymptomatic or mild, non-specific symptoms. Posterior cervical lympha-denopathy	Hydrocephalus, intracranial calcification, chorioretinitis. Jaundice, anemia, hepato-splenomegaly, lymphado-pathy

during pregnancy are the same as those found in nonpregnant women. *Escherichia coli* accounts for 80% to 90% of infections. Other Gram negative rods such as *Proteus mirabilis* and *Klebsiella pneumoniae* are also common. Enterococci, *Gardnerella vaginalis* and *Ureaplasma ureolyticum*, as well as Gram-positive organisms such as group B Streptococcus and *Staphylococcus saprophyticus* are less commonly found. Urethral catheterization contributes to increased risk of acquiring nosocomial UTIs.

SEXUALLY TRANSMITTED INFECTIONS

The Centers for Disease Control and Prevention (CDC) recommends screening for some sexually transmitted infections (STIs) at the first prenatal visit, and subsequently in the third trimester for mothers at high risk. Though sexually transmitted infections usually do not cause fevers in pregnancy, they may predispose to co-infections, and have implications for the fetus and neonate. Other screening tests that are recommended for all pregnant women include those for *Chlamydia trachomatis,* and women at risk should be tested for *Neisseria gonorrhea.* Women younger than 25 years and those who are at risk of *Chlamydia* (e.g., those who have multiple sex partners) should be rescreened in the third trimester. Women who continue to be at risk of gonorrhea should also be rescreened in the third trimester.

SKIN AND SOFT TISSUE INFECTIONS

The clinical presentation of skin and soft tissue infections in pregnancy is similar to that of nonpregnant patients. The extremities, buttocks, breasts, vulva or groin, and abdomen can be involved.

MENINGITIS

Meningitis is an inflammation of meninges, the membrane covering the brain and spinal cord. When a microorganism (usually a bacterium or virus) enters the subarachnoid space, there is inflammatory response in the meninges. The patient presents with headache, fever and daltered sensorium. Other features may include photophobia, vomiting, rash, and dehydration.

Bacterial meningitis is a medical emergency in which early diagnosis and treatment is imperative to prevent death and reduce long-term complications. Lumbar puncture is used to confirm the diagnosis in patients presenting with clinically suspected meningitis

PNEUMONIA

Pneumonia is the most frequent cause of non-obstetric infection in the pregnant patient and constitutes a serious complication of pregnancy. Depending on etiology, particular types of pneumonia can have very different implications for the pregnant woman, especially pneumonia of viral origin.

The clinical manifestations of acute bacterial pneumonia present with cough, fever, dyspnea, chills and sputum production being often the chief symptoms. Complications in the pregnant woman with pneumonia include anemia, empyema, bacteremia, and death. The most common pathogens in pregnancy are *Streptococcus pneumoniae, Haemophilus influenzae*, and *Mycoplasma pneumoniae.* Viral respiratory infections also can cause maternal pneumonia (about 5% of cases). Fungal pneumonias are rare in pregnancy. *Cryptococcus neoformans, Histoplasma capsulatum, Sporothrix schenckii, Blastomyces dermatitidis*, and *Coccidioides immitis* can cause pneumonia that is usually mild and self-limited disease. The atypical pneumonia syndrome with low-grade fever, gradual onset, mucoid sputum and patchy or interstitial infiltrates suggests infection with the atypical pneumonia pathogens.

PREVENTION OF INFECTION IN PREGNANCY

Like all adults and children, pregnant women are at risk for developing viral and bacterial infections. Infections are a particular concern during pregnancy since some infections are more severe in pregnant women or may harm the fetus or newborn. However, measures can be taken to minimize the chance of developing a potentially harmful illness during pregnancy.

Ideally, all women should consult their healthcare provider before conception. Pre-pregnancy testing for infections should include an assessment of rubella immunity, syphilis status, human immunodeficiency virus (HIV) status, and immunity to hepatitis B. Some countries test for varicella IgG antibody to exclude previous infection with chickenpox. Women in close contact with children, such as childcare workers, may be at increased risk of cytomegalovirus (CMV) infection during pregnancy, and should be tested for CMV IgG before conception.

A pre-pregnancy visit is also an opportunity to give dietary and other advice on how to reduce the risk of contracting Hepatitis E, listeriosis and toxoplasmosis
- Drink boiled water
- Avoid raw or undercooked meat and meat products

Diagnostic Modalities for Symptomatic Illness during Pregnancy

Clinical scenario	Probable diagnosis	Diagnostic tests
Influenza or glandular fever like illness (lethargy, fever, malaise, myalgia +/- headache, +/- lympha-denopathy)	Primary CMV infection	• *Tissue biopsy:* Presence of inclusion bodies (owl's eye) • IgG and IgM (paired sera)
	Primary toxoplasmosis	• Virus isolation from saliva, urine. • IgG and IgM (paired sera)
	Other viral infections	• Culture, serology where appropriate
Meningitis	Listeriosis	• Culture of feces, blood and/or urine and serology
Fever with rash, exposure	Rubella	• IgG & IgM (paired sera)
	Dengue	• Blood PCR (1–5 days) • Serum: NS1 antigen (2–7 days) • Serum: IgM antibody (> 7 days)
	Parvovirus infection	• IgG and IgM (paired sera)
	Enterovirus infection	• Throat swab or fecal culture
Vesicular rash	Varicella	• Swab from lesion: Demonstrate presence of multinucleated giant cells (Tzank smear) • Serology: IgG antibodies
	Hand, foot and mouth disease	• Throat swab and fecal culture
Any fever, dysuria (cystitis, pyelonephritis)	Urinary tract infection	• Urine microscopy, culture and antimicrobial susceptibility testing.
Genital lesions	Genital herpes	• HSV1 and HSV2 PCR • IgG and IgM (paired sera)
Vaginal discharge, diagnosis of other STI	Chlamydia, gonorrhoea	• *Cervical swab:* Gram stain, culture, serology and PCR • Check for syphilis, HBV and HIV serology
Abdominal pain	Chorioamnionitis	• Vaginal discharge: Gram stain and culture (for group B streptococci or abnormal vaginal flora associated with bacterial vaginosis)
Cough, dyspnea	Pneumonia	• Chest X-ray, sputum for stain and culture
Fever after returning from an endemic country	Malaria	• Peripheral blood smear • Rapid malaria antigen detection techniques (PfHPR-2) • Fluorescent staining • Malaria PCR
Fever after returning from an endemic country	Typhoid	• Antibody detection by widal test • Blood culture
Fever and abdominal pain, abnormal LFT's	Hepatitis	• ELISA for detection of HBsAg, HBeAg, anti-HBC and anti-HEV antibodies • Hepatitis B and C viral load

• Peel or wash raw fruit and vegetables thoroughly to remove contaminating soil

• Wash hands after disposing off cat litter or gardening.

Women who lack immunity to rubella, hepatitis B, or varicella, should be advised vaccination and pregnancy should be postponed for at least two months after completion of the vaccination. Routine antenatal screening generally should be offered to all pregnant women after obtaining informed consent. Other screening tests for sexually transmitted infections that are recommended for pregnant women include HIV, hepatitis B, syphilis, and *Chlamydia trachomatis*. Women at risk should be tested for *Neisseria gonorrhea* and hepatitis C.

Table 9.2: Immunization during pregnancy

Immunobiologic agent	Type of agent	Pregnancy Indications for immunization
Live virus vaccines		
Measles	Attenuated (Measles-Mumps-Rubella)	Contraindicated
Mumps	Attenuated	Contraindicated
Rubella	Attenuated	Contraindicated
Yellow fever	Attenuated	Contraindicated except if exposure is unavoidable
Varicella	Attenuated	Contraindicated
Poliomyelitis	Attenuated (oral, and enhanced potency inactivated)	Not routinely recommended, except women at increased risk of exposure
Other		
Influenza	Inactivated	All women in the 2nd and 3rd trimesters during the flu season; women at risk for pulmonary complications regardless of trimester
Hepatitis A	Inactivated	Pre- and post-exposure for at-risk women; international travellers
Hepatitis B	Recombinant purified surface antigen	Pre- and post-exposure for at-risk women
Inactivated Bacterial		
Typhoid	Killed or live attenuated	Except in exposure or travel to endemic areas
Pneumococcus	Polyvalent polysaccharide	In women with asplenia; metabolic, renal, cardiac, pulmonary disease; immunosuppressed; smokers
Meningococcal	Quadrivalent polysaccharide	Not altered by pregnancy
Toxoids		
Tetanus-diphtheria	Combined toxoids	Lack of primary series, or no booster within past 10 years

VACCINATION DURING PREGNANCY

Vaccines help keep a pregnant woman and her growing family healthy. The administration of vaccines during pregnancy poses a number of concerns to physicians and patients about the risk of transmitting a virus to a developing fetus. Live-virus vaccines are therefore generally contraindicated in pregnant women. Vaccines commonly administered by family physicians, and their indication for use during pregnancy, are as given in Table 9.2.

BIBLIOGRAPHY

1. Anantnarayan and Panikers's Textbook of Microbiology 9th edition.
2. www.antimicrobe.org/e42.asp
3. Gilbert GL. Infections in pregnant women. Med J Aust 2002;176(5):229–236.
4. Gilbert GL. Routine antenatal screening and prenatal diagnosis of vertically transmissible infection.
5. Hurley R. Fever and infectious diseases. 1995. In: de Swiet (ed) Medical disorders in obstetric practice. Blackwell Scientific Publications, Oxford. Baillieres Clin Obstet Gynaecol 1993;7:1–23.
6. Ledward RS, Ahmed BA. Viral infections in pregnancy. Update 1995; 42–48.
7. Maharaj D. Puerperal pyrexia: a review. Part I. Obstet Gynecol Surv 2007;62(6):393–399.
8. Maharaj D. Puerperal pyrexia: a review. Part II. Obstet Gynecol Surv 2007; 62(6):400–406.
9. Majeroni BA, Ukkadam S. Screening and Treatment for Sexually Transmitted Infections in Pregnancy. Am Fam Physician 2007;76(2):265–70.
10. www.cdc.gov/vaccines/pubs/preg-guide.htm

Non-infective Causes of Fever in Pregnancy

Ankesh R Sahetya, Divya Sahetya

INTRODUCTION

Besides the infectious causes of fever in pregnancy, the non-infectious causes of fever in pregnancy are hazardous to the successful outcome of pregnancy. The coexistence of pregnancy may aggravate the risk to maternal life of the more serious of these diseases. Mild exposures during the preimplantation period and more severe exposures during embryonic and fetal development often result in miscarriage, premature labor, growth restriction, and stillbirth.

SIGNIFICANCE OF FEVER IN PREGNANCY[2]

Studies have shown an increased risk of neural tube defects (NTD) in babies of women who had high temperatures early in pregnancy.[1] About 1 to 2 out of every 1,000 births has a neural tube defect. The most common type's being spina bifida and anencephaly. An opening in the spinal column is called spina bifida. A few studies have found a small increased risk for a heart defect, an abdominal wall defect, or an oral cleft when a fever occurs in early pregnancy, especially if the fever is untreated.

PATHOGENESIS[3]

The underlying sequence of events seems to be the removal of endotoxins from the circulation by fixed phagocytes of the reticuloendothelial system, followed by margination of polymorphonuclear leukocytes along the margins of the vessels. These two types of cells undergo activation to release endogenous pyrogen into the circulation. The pyrogen produced in response to toxic, immunological or infectious stimuli, is induced through the release of lymphocytic lymphokines arising in response to antigenic recognition, and acts on the hypothalamic thermoregulatory center, transmitting information to the vasomotor center, possibly through production of prostaglandins.

ETIOLOGY[3]

Neoplasms	Connective tissue disorders	Other
Lymphoma	Rheumatic fever	Drug fever
Leukaemia	Systemic lupus erythematosis	Thromboembolism
Melanoma	Rheumatoid arthritis	Sarcoidosis
Metastasis		Hemolytic anemia
Retro peritoneal sarcoma		
Tumours of lung, kidney, pancreas, liver		

LYMPHOMA

Hodgkin's lymphoma is a cancer that develops in the lymph system, part of the body's immune system. Hodgkin's lymphoma in pregnant women is the same as the disease in nonpregnant women of childbearing age.[4] However, treatment is different for pregnant women.

CLINICAL FEATURES

- Painless, swollen lymph nodes in the neck, underarm, or groin.
- Fevers for no known reason.
- Drenching night sweats.
- Weight loss for no known reason.
- Itchy skin.
- Feeling very tired.

INVESTIGATIONS

- Complete blood count
- Erythrocyte sedimentation rate
- Lymph node biopsy
- Immunophenotyping

TREATMENT[4]

The prognosis (chance of recovery) depends on the stage of the cancer (the number of lymph node groups affected and the number of places outside of the lymph nodes to which the cancer has spread). Most pregnant patients with newly diagnosed Hodgkin's lymphoma can be cured.

Treatment options depend on the following:
- The stage of the cancer.
- The patient's symptoms and general health.
- The wishes of the patient.
- The age of the fetus.

After Hodgkin's lymphoma during pregnancy has been diagnosed, tests are done to find out if cancer cells have spread within the lymph system or to other parts of the body.

To protect the fetus from the harms of radiation, tests that do not use radiation are used in the staging process. These include:
- *MRI (magnetic resonance imaging):* A procedure that uses a magnet, radio waves, and a computer to make a series of detailed pictures of areas inside the body. This procedure is also called nuclear magnetic resonance imaging (NMRI).
- *Ultrasound exam:* A procedure in which high-energy sound waves (ultrasound) are bounced off internal tissues or organs and make echoes. The echoes form a picture of body tissues called a sonogram.

STAGES OF HODGKIN'S LYMPHOMA DURING PREGNANCY MAY INCLUDE A, B, E, AND S[5]

- *A:* The patient has no symptoms.
- *B:* The patient has symptoms such as fever, weight loss, or night sweats.
- *E:* "E" stands for extranodal and means the cancer is found in an area or organ other than the lymph nodes or has spread to tissues beyond, but near, the major lymphatic areas.
- *S:* "S" stands for spleen and means the cancer is found in the spleen.

Treatment Options[4]

Different types of treatment are available for pregnant patients with Hodgkin's lymphoma. Treatment is carefully chosen to protect the fetus. Treatment decisions are based on the mother's wishes, the stage of the Hodgkin's lymphoma, and the age of the fetus. The treatment plan may change as the symptoms, cancer, and pregnancy change. Choosing the most appropriate cancer treatment is a decision that ideally involves the patient, family, and healthcare team.

Radiation Therapy

The way the radiation therapy is given depends on the type and stage of the cancer being treated.

To avoid any risk to the fetus, radiation therapy should be postponed until after delivery, if possible. If immediate treatment is needed, pregnant women with Hodgkin's lymphoma may decide to continue the pregnancy and receive radiation therapy. However, lead used to shield the fetus may not protect it from scattered radiation that could possibly cause cancer in the future.

Chemotherapy

The fetus cannot be protected from being exposed to chemotherapy when the mother is treated. Some chemotherapy regimens may cause birth defects when given in the first trimester. Vinblastine is an anticancer drug that has not been linked with birth defects in the second half of pregnancy.

Watchful waiting is closely monitoring a patient's condition without giving any treatment unless symptoms appear or change. Delivery may be induced when the fetus is 32 to 36 weeks old, so that the mother can begin treatment.

Steroid Therapy

Certain steroid drugs have been found to help chemotherapy work better and help stop the growth of cancer cells. Steroids can also help the lungs of the fetus develop faster than normal. This is important when delivery is induced early.

HODGKIN'S LYMPHOMA DURING THE FIRST TRIMESTER OF PREGNANCY

When Hodgkin's lymphoma is diagnosed in the first trimester of pregnancy, it does not necessarily mean that the patient will be advised to end the pregnancy. Each patient's treatment will depend on the stage of the lymphoma, how fast it is growing, and the patient's wishes. For women who choose to continue the pregnancy, treatment of Hodgkin's lymphoma during the first trimester of pregnancy may include the following:

• Watchful waiting when the cancer is above the diaphragm and is slow-growing.

Delivery may be induced when the fetus is 32 to 36 weeks old so the mother can begin treatment.
• Radiation therapy above the diaphragm, with the fetus shielded.
• Systemic chemotherapy using one or more drugs.

HODGKIN'S LYMPHOMA DURING THE SECOND HALF OF PREGNANCY

When Hodgkin's lymphoma is diagnosed in the second half of pregnancy, most patients can delay treatment until after the baby is born. Treatment of Hodgkin's lymphoma during the second half of pregnancy may include the following:

• Watchful waiting, with plans to induce delivery when the fetus is 32 to 36 weeks old.
• Systemic chemotherapy using one or more drugs.
• Steroid therapy.
• Radiation therapy to relieve breathing problems caused by a large tumor in the chest.

LEUKAEMIA

Leukemia in pregnancy remains a challenging therapeutic prospect. The prevalence is low at ~1 in 10000 pregnancies. The management of the leukemias in pregnancy requires close collaboration with obstetric and neonatology colleagues as both the maternal and fetal outcomes must be taken into consideration.[6] The decision to introduce or delay chemotherapy must be balanced against the impact on maternal and fetal survival and morbidity. Invariably, acute leukemia diagnosed in the first trimester necessitates intensive chemotherapy that is likely to induce fetal malformations. As delaying treatment in this situation is usually inappropriate, counseling with regard to termination of pregnancy is often essential.

Acute Leukemia

The presentation of acute leukemia in pregnancy is broadly similar to the non-pregnant state, although pregnancy may obscure some of the clinical signs. The majority of the leukemias diagnosed in pregnancy are acute and predominantly myeloid as the incidence of acute lymphoblastic leukemia is more common in childhood and adolescence. If the disease is left untreated, it will likely result in maternal and fetal mortality and a decision to delay start of induction chemotherapy negatively impacts on the likelihood of remission. The therapeutic approach to the management of acute leukemias in pregnancy regardless of subtype is generally similar. Although a bone marrow aspirate and trephine biopsy may be performed safely in pregnancy, these can be avoided if confirmation is clearly possible by means of peripheral blood microscopy, flow cytometry and molecular analysis.

Acute Myeloid Leukaemia

AML occurs more frequently with advancing age and as expected, there is a greater body of data regarding the therapeutic approach for AML in pregnancy. Due to the aggressive nature of the disease, treatment cannot be delayed indefinitely and the balance between the consequences of intensive chemotherapy on both fetus and mother, as well as the effect of postponing treatment on the mother, must be carefully evaluated.

First Trimester

Developmental effects on the fetus are dependent on the point in gestation at which chemotherapy is given. Damage to the majority of the cells of the conceptus is likely to result in miscarriage. End-organ damage (heart, neural tube, and limbs) is induced by chemotherapy during this time, the effects are likely to be irreversible. As a result, chemotherapy administered within the first trimester is associated with the greatest risk of miscarriage, fetal death and congenital malformation, ranging from 10% to 20%. Chemotherapy also inhibits trophoblast migration and proliferation, which may contribute to neonatal low birth weight.

Second and Third Trimesters

The risk of fetal malformation is generally accepted to reduce as the pregnancy advances. Exposure to chemotherapy after the first trimester results in an increased incidence of intrauterine growth retardation (which is also affected by maternal nutritional status throughout), preterm delivery, and fetal death, but no increase in the incidence of congenital abnormalities and in particular no documented rise in childhood malignancy or unfavorable neurological development even though the latter continues throughout gestation. Treatment during the third trimester generally results in the least complications; however there is minor risk of pancytopenia immediately prior to delivery. Early delivery may be considered if the leukemia presents sufficiently late in pregnancy. If chemotherapy is considered mandatory, then it is important to anticipate the myelosuppressive effects of chemotherapy on the fetus and plan supportive care following delivery which should be timed if possible to coincide with recovery of the maternal blood count.

Supportive Care

A number of additional supportive agents are usually used to ensure that the chemotherapy is well tolerated, including antiemetic, commonly ondansetron and metoclopramide as these appear safe in pregnancy.

Chronic Leukemias

Chronic Myeloid Leukemia[7]

Chronic myeloid leukemia (CML) accounts for 15% of adult leukemias, but only a small proportion of patients are diagnosed during childbearing age as the median age at diagnosis is in the sixth decade. CML occurs in up to 10% of pregnancy-associated leukemias, with an annual incidence of 1 per 100000 pregnancies.

For a patient presenting with chronic myeloid leukaemia in chronic phase in the first trimester, treatment is probably unnecessary if the white cell count remains below $100 \times 10^9/L$ and the platelet count is $<500 \times 10^9/L$.

Leukapheresis is recommended to maintain a threshold below these levels. The frequency of leukapheresis will naturally be tailored to the individual and vary according to the gestation, but in general can be performed as often as alternate days to 1 to 2 weekly. Low-molecular weight heparin as well as aspirin can be used once platelets exceed $1000 \times 10^9/L$. For women who are leukapheresis intolerant or for whom it proves ineffective, IFN-α is an option after the second trimester.

Management of Pregnancy while on Treatment[6]

With first- and/or second-generation tyrosine kinase inhibitors (TKI), most patients will achieve deep and durable responses, consistent with a normal life expectancy. As a consequence, many women are seeking advice regarding the feasibility and safety of becoming pregnant while on treatment. Because observed congenital abnormalities have occurred with the use of TKI in the first trimester, patients should be advised to discontinue treatment before conception. Confidence in withdrawing imatinib has been gained from "stopping imatinib" studies which show that roughly 40% of patients continue to maintain a deep response with undetectable BCR-ABL1 transcripts when imatinib has been discontinued after the achievement of a complete molecular response (CMR) for a period of 2 years.

Chronic Lymphocytic Leukemia

The incidence is very rare. Therapeutic options include leukapheresis chlorambucil, and more recently rituximab, a chimeric anti-CD20 monoclonal B-cell-depleting antibody. Although chlorambucil is embryotoxic (neural tube defects, skeletal and renal abnormalities), successful outcomes in pregnancy have been reported despite chlorambucil exposure in the first trimester. The assessment of rituximab exposure during pregnancy has been confounded by concomitant chemotherapy use, and although a few congenital malforma-tions or neonatal infections have ensued, women should continue to avoid pregnancy for ≥12 months after rituximab exposure until more definitive data are available.

LIPOSARCOMA IN PREGNANCY

Liposarcoma during pregnancy is extremely rare and often discovered incidentally by abdominal or pelvic ultrasound exam. The most common clinical feature is an asympto-matic palpable mass, which often is hidden and confused by the pregnancy itself.[8] The second most common symptom is pain, such as abdominal pain or pelvic pain.[9]

Complete surgical resection of the tumor is the best choice of treatment, but an individualized approach should be taken, according to gestational age, tumor location, fetus status and the patient's general condition. The effects of additional chemo-therapy or radiotherapy after surgery are still controversial.

CONNECTIVE TISSUE DISORDERS IN PREGNANCY

Connective tissue is the structure that holds the body together and is composed largely of collagen and elastin. Connective tissue disorders are classified into a number of groups. The significance of pregnancy varies considerably according to the type of the disease:

- Hereditary connective tissue disorders (HCTDs) includes such diseases as Ehlers-Danlos syndrome, Marfan's syndrome and pseudoxanthoma elasticum (PXE).
- Mixed connective tissue disease (MCTD).
- This was initially considered as an overlap or combination of systemic lupus erythematosus (SLE), scleroderma, and polymyositis.
- Patients have features of each of these three diseases. Typically, they also have very high titres of antinuclear antibodies (ANAs) and antibodies to ribonucleoprotein (anti-RNP).

The hereditary forms tend to manifest fairly early in life. They are not often apparent at birth but are usually diagnosed before the advent of reproduction. The autoimmune forms tend to present after the reproductive years but it is not at all uncommon for them to present before middle age. Reproductive problems may be the presenting feature.

Epidemiology

- The HCTDs are usually inherited in a typical Mendelian form as autosomal dominant. Males and females are equally affected.
- The autoimmune diseases are acquired rather than inherited but they do tend to run in families. The exact aetiology is uncertain but if there is an external trigger, it would appear that a genetic predisposition is involved.
- The conditions are more common in women.

Pregnancy in Hereditary Connective Tissue Disorders

For the hereditary forms, genetic counselling is important, ideally before the woman becomes pregnant.

EHLERS-DANLOS SYNDROME

The risk varies considerably according to the type of the condition:

- Obstetric complications include risk of uterine rupture during labour, damage to the vagina and perineum, bleeding and rupture of blood vessels and the colon during the puerperium.[10]
- In type IV there is a risk for severe bleeding and vessel rupture associated with pregnancy.[11]
- In type II a Shirodkar's suture may be required to treat cervical incompetence.
- Generally Ehlers-Danlos syndrome is well tolerated in pregnancy except for type IV.

MARFAN'S SYNDROME

- The major risk for women with Marfan's syndrome is aortic dissection in pregnancy. Family history may indicate the level of this risk but echocardiography to assess the aortic root in pregnancy should be used.
- Aortic dissection is not the only problem and a multidisciplinary approach is recommended.[12]
- Surgery may be required before embarking on pregnancy. Aortic repair can be performed during pregnancy.
- Beta-blockers may be protective although they are associated with the risk of low birth-weight babies.

Pregnancy in Autoimmune Connective Tissue Disorders

As well as any effects caused directly by the connective tissue disorder, the woman may be taking drugs for the condition and these may be teratogenic, e.g. methotrexate which induces abortion. The relative risks and benefits of the various drugs in pregnancy need to be carefully weighed.

Systemic Lupus Erythematosus

In women with SLE the acronym **'PATH'** represents:

- **P**roteinuria.
- **A**ntiphospholipid syndrome.

- **T**hrombocytopenia.
- **H**ypertension early in pregnancy.

All of these are serious risk factors for adverse pregnancy outcomes.[13]

Pregnancy in Patients with Systemic Lupus Erythematosus

Fertility is normal and pregnancy is safe in mild or stable SLE. In severe SLE, pregnancy should be delayed until the disease is better controlled. *See* also the separate article on *Systemic Lupus Erythematosus*.

Effects on Fertility

- Women with rheumatoid arthritis (RA) have fewer children than average but this appears to be a conscious decision related to the difficulty of rearing children, with the limitations of the disease, rather than problems of fecundity.[8]
- However, a survey of American women with SLE and RA found that:[9]
    - Hypertensive disorders of pregnancy occurred in 23.2% of those with SLE and 11.1% of those with RA compared with 7.8% of the general population.
    - They tended to have more caesarean sections and longer stay in hospital.
    - They also tended to be older than the general population having babies but this did not account for the difference.
- In women with stable SLE, the use of oral contraceptives does not increase the risk of flare-up.[10]

RENAL CELL CARCINOMA IN PREGNANCY

Renal cell carcinoma accounts for 3% of all adult malignancies, it is rare in women of childbearing age. To date there are reports of about fifty cases diagnosed during pregnancy. It is the most common renal neoplasm reported in pregnancy, accounting for half of all primary tumours.[14] Sex and age matched data do not exist to allow comparison of the relative proportion occurring outside of pregnancy, although in general terms there is no evidence of an increased incidence of malignant neoplasms in pregnancy.

Clinical Features

The commonest presenting symptoms of such tumours were:
- Palpable mass (88%)
- Pain (50%)
- Hematuria
- Hypertension
- Diagnosis

Investigations

Diagnostic evaluation of the pregnant patient with possible renal carcinoma requires special consideration of non-invasive techniques and as little radiation exposure as possible to mother and fetus.

1. As a first step, urine should be sent for cytological analysis.

    In non-pregnant patients intravenous pyelography (IVP) and abdominal CT are the modalities frequently employed in the evaluation of renal tumours, but there is no proven safe threshold dose of radiation exposure to the fetus.

2. Abdominal ultrasound along with magnetic resonance imaging (MRI) can adequately identify, differentiate between, and stage solid renal masses in most cases, and with their avoidance of radiation exposure to the fetus these are the investigations of choice.

    Such cases should be managed in a multidisciplinary setting involving urologists, obstetricians, neonatologists, radiologists, histopathologists and oncologists.

Treatment

The standard surgical treatment of most stages of renal cell carcinoma is a radical nephrectomy, involving the en bloc removal of the entire kidney and perinephric fat within

Gerota's fascia. This has been performed via both transperitoneal and extraperitoneal approaches. The small numbers of reported cases of renal cell carcinoma in pregnancy allow a few conclusions to be drawn regarding the outcomes of each. However, avoidance of disruption of the peritoneal cavity in the extraperitoneal approach may theoretically be associated with less uterine irritation and in turn fewer obstetric complications, including preterm labour.

THROMBOEMBOLISM IN PREGNANCY

Venous thromboembolism (VTE) refers to the formation of a thrombus within veins. This can occur anywhere in the venous system but the clinically predominant sites are in the vessels of the leg [giving rise to deep vein thrombosis (DVT)] and in the lungs [resulting in a pulmonary embolus (PE)].

The pathophysiology of VTE in pregnancy appears to relate to the increased venous stasis noted during this period but other factors such as alterations in the balance of proteins of the coagulation and fibrinolytic systems have also been implicated.[15]

Epidemiology

- VTE affects about 1 in 100,000 women of childbearing age.[16]

- It is up to 10 times more common in pregnant than in non-pregnant women of a similar age.
- It occurs in about 1/1,000 pregnancies in women under the age of 35.[15]
- It occurs in 2.4/1,000 pregnancies in women over the age of 35.
- Inherited thrombophilia is present in 30–50% of women with pregnancy-associated VTE.[16]
- 10–20% of VTEs are PEs which are the main contributors to VTE mortality.
- Mortality rate

Thrombosis and thromboembolism was the leading cause of maternal deaths between 2010–2012 in the UK, occurring in 1.08 in 100,000 maternities.[17]

- 62% of women with fatal VTEs die in the first trimester although the risk per day is actually greatest in the weeks following delivery.
- 71% of postpartum deaths from VTE occur following vaginal delivery.
- 10% of postpartum deaths from VTE occur following operative (interventional) vaginal delivery.

Risk Factors[18]

There are a number of known risk factors, some hereditary and others acquired and in

Inherited factors	Acquired factors	Factors specific to pregnancy[16]
Factor V Leiden mutation (most common)	Obesity—body mass index (BMI) ≥ 30 kg/m^2	Venous stasis
Prothrombin gene G20210A mutation	Immobilisation (> 4 days of bed rest)	Maternal age of ≥ 35 years
Antithrombin III deficiency	Previous thrombotic event	Multiparity
Protein C deficiency	Trauma	Gestation < 36 weeks
Protein S deficiency	Inflammatory bowel disease	Instrument-assisted or caesarean delivery
Hyperhomocysteinaemia	Cancer	Hemorrhage
Disorders of plasminogen and plasminogen activation	Oestrogen therapy (including contraception and hormone replacement therapy)	Pre-eclampsia
Strong family history	Antiphospholipid syndrome	Prolonged labor
Dysfibrinogenaemia	Gross varicose veins	Sepsis, including urinary tract infections
	Nephrotic syndrome	

80% of patients, at least one risk factor can be identified. Notably, the antenatal period is known to be a weak risk factor and the postpartum period a moderate risk factor.

Often more than one risk factor is present and these should be actively identified when assessing the patient for VTE during and post-pregnancy.

Presentation

- *DVT:* Leg pain and discomfort (the left is more commonly affected), swelling, tenderness, oedema, increased temperature and a raised white cell count. There may also be abdominal pain. The difficulty is that some of these symptoms may be found in normal pregnancies. The patient may also be asymptomatic with a retrospective diagnosis being made following a PE.

- *PE:* Dyspnoea, pleuritic chest pain, haemoptysis, faintness, collapse. The patient may have focal signs in the chest, tachypnoea, a raised jugular venous pressure (JVP) and there may be ECG changes (S1Q3T3). Arterial blood gases taken with the patient sitting down may show respiratory alkalosis and hypoxaemia. There may also be symptoms or signs of a DVT.

Investigations and Diagnosis

Any woman with symptoms and signs suggestive of VTE should have objective testing performed promptly. Treatment with low molecular weight heparin (LMWH) should be started immediately (before diagnosis), unless treatment is strongly contraindicated. Many hospitals have local policies regarding the management of these patients. This may involve the obstetricians, haematologists, physicians and radiologists.

Deep Venous Thrombosis

If there is a clinical suspicion of a DVT, arrange an urgent compression duplex ultrasound scan. If this is negative and your suspicion is low, discontinue treatment. If it is negative but your suspicion is high, repeat the scan (or order an alternative imaging modality) one week later, whilst keeping the patient anticoagulated. If this is negative, discontinue anticoagulation.

Pulmonary Embolism

If there is a clinical suspicion of a PE, organize a CXR and if this is normal, arrange compression duplex Doppler. The CXR may identify other pulmonary disease, such as pneumonia, pneumothorax or lobar collapse. If these are negative, the patient needs to have a ventilation-perfusion (V/Q) lung scan or a computed tomography pulmonary angiogram (CTPA)—discuss with the radiologist.

Blood Tests[16]

- Complete blood count
- Liver function tests
- Serum Fibrinogen
- Activated partial thromboplastin time
- Fibrin degradation products
- D-dimer is an unreliable test to carry out in these patients. In pregnancy, it can be elevated because of the physiological changes in the coagulation system and levels become 'abnormal' at term and in the postnatal period in most healthy pregnant women.

Management

General Points

- In a woman with a past history of VTE or with a known inherited thrombophilia, it is best to refer her prior to a planned pregnancy for optimum prophylaxis throughout the pregnancy.[16] Refer all women who are on warfarin, as this will have to be stopped or replaced by heparin before the seventh week of conception, depending on her risk of VTE.

- Medical anticoagulation is the treatment of choice for acute VTE. Subsequently, surgical interventions may be considered: patients suffering from recurrent PEs despite adequate anticoagulation (or where there is an absolute contra-indication to anticoagulation) may benefit from placement of a temporary caval filter and, in those cases where there is limb or life-threatening embolus, a surgical embo-lectomy or thrombus fragmentation may be attempted.[18]
- Anticoagulation is by far the most common treatment option. Heparin is the most frequently used drug, being non-toxic to the fetus (it does not cross the placental barrier). However, its main disadvantages are that it has to be parentally administered and, in the long-term, may give rise to heparin-induced osteoporosis and thrombocytopenia. Warfarin is the other treatment option in the postnatal patient but it must be avoided antenatally, as it is teratogenic and can also cause placental abruption and fetal/neonatal hemorrhage.
- In clinically suspected DVT or PE, treatment with unfractionated heparin or LMWH should be given until the diagnosis is excluded by objective testing, unless treatment is strongly contraindicated.

Initiating Treatment[19]

There are several different types of heparin to choose from:
- *LMWH:* This is the drug of choice. It has been shown to be more effective than unfractionated heparin with lower mortality and fewer hemorrhagic complica-tions in the initial treatment of DVT in non-pregnant subjects. LMWHs are as effective as unfractionated heparin for treatment of PE. The exact dose will depend on patient's early pregnancy weight and should be administered subcutaneously twice daily. There should be clear local guidelines for the dosage of LMWH to be used.

- Intravenous unfractionated heparin: This is an extensively used drug in the acute management of VTE, particularly massive PE with cardiovascular compromise. It is initiated with a loading dose of 5,000 international units (IU) followed by a continuous infusion of 1,000–2,000 IU/hour depending on activated partial thrombo-plastin time (aPTT) measurements (daily at least), the first of which is taken six hours after the loading dose. Subcutaneous unfractionated heparin: This has been shown to be as effective as the intravenous form. It is administered as a 5,000 IU bolus and subsequent 15,000–20,000 IU doses at 12-hourly intervals. The aPTT needs to be checked and is best done midway between the 12-hourly doses, once every 24 hours. A target of 1.5–2.5 times the control should be aimed for.

Additionally, the leg should be elevated and a graduated elastic compression stocking applied to reduce oedema. Mobilisation with graduated elastic compression stockings should be encouraged.

Maintenance Therapy

During Pregnancy

Heparins are the maintenance treatment of choice. Dose-adjusted subcutaneous, un-fractionated heparin or subcutaneous LMWH are effective alternatives to oral anticoagulants in maintenance treatment of VTE.
- Subcutaneous LMWH appears to have advantages over aPTT-monitored unfrac-tionated heparin in the maintenance treatment of VTE in pregnancy. The simplified therapeutic regimen for LMWH tends to be more convenient for patients, minimising blood tests (routine platelet counts are not required and levels of anti-Xa will only need to be monitored where there are extremes of weight: <50 kg or >90 kg) and allowing outpatient treatment. Women should be taught to self-inject and can then be managed as outpatients until delivery.

- If unfractionated heparin is used, monitor the platelet count at least every other day for the first 14 days or until treatment is stopped (whichever comes first).

Seek specialist advice if the patient develops heparin-induced thrombocytopenia or a heparin allergy and requires continuing anticoagulant therapy. She should be managed with the heparinoid, danaparoid sodium or fondaparinux, under specialist supervision.

Labor

When the patient thinks she is going into labor, she should stop injecting and get in touch with the delivery ward staff who will manage the anticoagulation throughout labor and immediately post-delivery. Alternatively, planned elective induction of labor or cesarean section at least 12 hours after prophylactic-dose LMWH or 24 hours after therapeutic-dose LMWH can be considered.[16] As these patients are at high risk of hemorrhage, they will be managed with intravenous unfractionated heparin throughout this time. Regional anaesthetic or analgesic techniques should not be undertaken until at least 24 hours after the last dose of therapeutic LMWH.

Postpartum Period

Depending on the patient's individual circumstances, she may be managed with ongoing heparin treatment or warfarin postpartum. If she opts for warfarin, this needs to be avoided until at least day three postpartum with an INR check at day two of warfarin treatment: Aim for an INR between 2 and 3. Continue heparin treatment until there have been two successive readings of an INR > 2.16.

Postnatal review for women who develop VTE during pregnancy or the puerperium should, whenever possible, be at an obstetric medicine clinic or a joint obstetric haematology clinic.

Stopping Treatment

In theory, therapy should be continued for six months as would be the case for non-pregnant patients. However, the postpartum state is a period of physiological fluctuation of coagulation factors. Therefore, current advice is to continue therapy for at least 6–12 weeks postpartum or until at least three months of therapy have been completed.

Complications

- Fetal loss
- Intrauterine growth restriction:
- *HELLP syndrome:* Haemolysis, Elevated Liver enzymes, Low Platelet count—this may be associated with certain forms of thrombophilia.

POST-THROMBOTIC SYNDROME

Up to 60% of patients who have experienced a DVT go on to have post-thrombotic syndrome up to 12 months following the acute event. This arises from damage to the lumen of the vein following the presence of a thrombus. Subsequently, patients manifest symptoms and signs akin to those of varicose veins: Aching, swollen legs, pruritus, dermatitis and hyperpigmentation of the affected area. Ulceration and cellulitis may complicate the picture. Compression stockings worn on the affected leg for at least two years have been recommended after the acute event to reduce the risk of developing post-thrombotic syndrome.

Other Complications

Prolonged unfractionated heparin use during pregnancy may result in osteoporosis and fractures.

RCOG GUIDELINES
Antenatal

Regardless of their VTE risk, dehydration and immobilisation of the patient should be avoided throughout pregnancy.

- Women at high risk of VTE in pregnancy should be offered pre-pregnancy counselling and a prospective management plan for thromboprophylaxis in pregnancy. All women with previous VTE should receive postpartum prophylaxis, as this is the time of highest risk.
- In addition, women whose original VTE was unprovoked, idiopathic or related to oestrogen, or who have other risk factors, a family history of VTE in a first-degree relative or a documented thrombophilia require LMWH antenatally and for six weeks postpartum.
- Women with recurrent VTE may already be on warfarin. They should be advised to stop warfarin and change to LMWH as soon as pregnancy is confirmed, ideally within two weeks of the missed period and before the sixth week of pregnancy. Women not on warfarin should be advised to start LMWH as soon as they have a positive pregnancy test.
- Women with asymptomatic inherited or acquired thrombophilia only, may be managed with close surveillance antenatally and be considered for LMWH for at least seven days postpartum. Exceptions are women with antithrombin deficiency, those with more than one thrombophilic defect (including homozygosity for factor V Leiden) or those with additional risk factors where antenatal prophylaxis should be considered.

Intrapartum

Women taking LMWH should be advised that, if they bleed vaginally or contractions begin, they should not inject any further doses. They should be assessed in hospital and further doses be prescribed by medical staff.

Postpartum

- All women with obesity (BMI greater than 40 kg/m^2) should be considered for prophylactic LMWH for seven days after delivery. Other postnatal risks include prolonged labor, immobility, infection, hemorrhage and blood transfusion.
- All women who have had an emergency caesarean section should be considered for LMWH for seven days after delivery. All women who have had an elective caesarean section who have one or more additional risk factors should be considered for LMWH for seven days after delivery.

In addition, properly applied graduated compression stockings are recommended for women travelling long-distance for more than four hours, women who are still outpatients but have prior VTE (usually combined with LMWH), women who are hospitalized and have a contraindication to LMWH and those who are hospitalised post-cesarean section (combined with LMWH) and considered to be at particularly high risk of VTE.

Key points for practice

- Venous thromboembolism is a very important non-infective cause of fever which can be prevented by prophylaxis in antenatal and postnatal period for patients at high risk.
- Malignancies although a very rare cause of fever in pregnancy, should always be kept in the back of the mind.
- Rare causes like lymphoma and leukemia, can be lethal if not dealt with promptly.
- Retroperitoneal and other pelvic causes although rare can be ruled out by ultrasonography early in pregnancy.

REFERENCES

1. Wang M1, Wang ZP, Gong R, Zhao ZT; 'Maternal flu or fever, medications use in the first trimester and the risk for neural tube defects: A hospital-based case-control study in China', ChildsNerv Syst. 2014 Apr;30(4):665–71. doi: 10.1007/s00381-013-2305-3. Epub 2013 Oct 26.
2. Botto LD, et al. 2013. National Birth Defects Prevention Study. Congenital heart defects after maternal fever. Am J Obstet Gynecol. 210(4):359. e1-359.e11.

3. Chambers CD, et al. 1998. Maternal fever and birth outcome: A prospective study. Teratology. 58:251–257.

4. Eyre TA, Lau IJ, Mackillop L, Collins GP, "Management and controversies of classical Hodgkin lymphoma in pregnancy", Br J Haematol. 2015 Feb 13.doi: 10.1111/bjh.13327.

5. Dam Lv, Han SN, Dierickx D, Amant F, "Optimal staging of lymphoma during pregnancy is crucial", Womens Health (LondEngl). 2015 Mar;11(2):101–2. doi: 10.2217/whe.14.77.

6. Palani R, Milojkovic D, Apperley JF, "Managing pregnancy in chronic myeloid leukaemia", Ann Hematol. 2015 Apr;94Suppl 2:167-76. doi: 10.1007/s00277-015-2317-z. Epub 2015 Mar 27.

7. Agarwal K, Patel M, Agarwal V, A Complicated Case of Acute Promyelocytic Leukemia in the Second Trimester of Pregnancy Successfully Treated with All-trans-Retinoic Acid. Case Rep Hematol. 2015;2015:634252. doi: 10.1155/2015/634252. Epub 2015 Mar 5.

8. Enzinger FM, Weiss SW. Soft tissue tumors. 3rd ed. St Louis: Mosby; 1995.

9. Boulay R, Podczaski E. Ovarian cancer complicating pregnancy. ObstetGynecolClin North Am.1998;25:385–399.

10. Erez Y, Ezra Y, Rojansky N; Ehlers-Danlos type IV in pregnancy. A case report and a literature review. Fetal DiagnTher. 2008;23(1):7–9. Epub 2007 Oct 9.

11. Combeer EL, Combeer AD; A rare cause of maternal death: liver and inferior vena cava rupture due to Eur J Anaesthesiol. 2008 Sep;25(9):765–7. Epub 2008 Apr 10.

12. Bowater SE, Thorne SA; Management of pregnancy in women with acquired and congenital heart disease. Postgrad Med J. 2010 Feb;86(1012):100–5.

13. Clowse ME, Magder LS, Witter F, et al; Early risk factors for pregnancy loss in lupus. Obstet Gynecol. 2006 Feb;107(2 Pt 1):293–9.

14. Walker JL, Knight EL. Renal cell carcinoma in pregnancy. Cancer 1986;58: 2343–7.

15. James AH; Venous thromboembolism in pregnancy. ArteriosclerThrombVasc Biol. 2009 Mar;29(3):326–31. doi: 10.1161/ATVBAHA. 109.184127.

16. Lim W, Eikelboom JW, Ginsberg JS; Inherited thrombophilia and pregnancy associated venous thromboembolism. BMJ. 2007 Jun 23;334(7607): 1318–21.

17. Saving Lives, Improving Mothers' Care - Lessons learned to inform future maternity care from the UK and Ireland Confidential Enquiries into Maternal Deaths and Morbidity 2009–2012; MBRACE-UK, Dec 2014.

18. Condliffe R, Elliot CA, Hughes RJ, et al; Management dilemmas in acute pulmonary embolism. Thorax. 2014 Feb;69(2):174–80. doi: 10.1136/thoraxjnl-2013-204667. Epub 2013 Dec.

19. British National Formulary; NICE Evidence Services.

11

Monsoon Fevers in Pregnancy

Aditya Gupta, Niteen D Karnik

INTRODUCTION

Monsoon sees a spurt in various water borne and vector borne diseases. These diseases are more dangerous when they affect pregnant females. During pregnancy a multi-factorial suppression of cell mediated immunity aimed at protecting the fetus from the mother has been reported. Various theories like decreased lymphocytic proliferative response, decreased natural killer cell activity have been proposed.

Management of infections during pregnancy is challenging considering the fact that infections as well as their treatment can adversely affect the mother, fetus and the pregnancy outcome. The infections commonly seen in pregnancy during monsoon are as follows: malaria, dengue, leptospirosis, hepatitis E, typhoid. In addition, physician has to be alert to possibility of a spill over from seasonal fevers like swine flu.

MALARIA

Malaria infection during pregnancy is a significant public health problem. It is associated with anemia, an increased risk of severe malaria, and may lead to spontaneous abortion, stillbirth, prematurity and low birth weight. The complications and mortality are not exclusive to *P. falciparum* malaria and are also seen with *P. vivax* malaria.[1]

Clinical Features

Uncomplicated malaria is characterized by a cold stage, consisting of cold sensation and shivering, and a hot stage, with fever, headache, sweating. Symptoms generally last for 6 to 10 hours and occur every 2 to 3 days, depending on the infecting species. However, this classical paroxysm may be modified in patients with subclinical immunity. Fever may be mild with anemia, mild jaundice and splenomegaly may be present. Also there is intense accumulation of parasitized RBCs in placental microcirculation which adds to anemia. Interestingly, the greatest degree of placental infestation is seen in women who have the highest level of immunity, leading to milder maternal symptoms and a disproportionate increase in fetal compli-cations.[2]

The criteria for severe malaria are outlined in Table 11.1.[3]

The complications of severe malaria in pregnancy are outlined in Table 11.2.[3,4] Certain specific presentations[3,4] are discussed below.

Malaria with Anemia in Pregnancy

- Normochromic Normocytic anemia
- Needs blood transfusion if Hb <7gm/dl or PCV < 20%
- If infestation rate is high (>5%), rapid fall in Hb occurs on treatment due to lysis of parasitized RBCs.

Table 11.1: Criteria for severe malaria[3]

1. Cerebral malaria, defined as unarousable coma not attributable to any other cause in a patient with falciparum malaria. It includes
    a. Altered sensorium, convulsions, comab.
    b. Retinal hemorrhages, papilledemac.
    c. Eye movement abnormalities, dysconjugate gazed.
    d. Mild neck stiffness, pouting, bruxism but no neck rigidity.
    e. Bilateral UMN signs
    f. Decorticate and decerebrate rigidity
    g. CSF studies—increased CSF pressure and proteins, cells up to 10 WBCs /μl
2. Severe normocytic anemia.
3. Hypoglycemia.
4. Metabolic acidosis with respiratory distress.
5. Fluid and electrolyte disturbances.
6. Acute renal failure.
7. Acute pulmonary oedema and acute respiratory distress syndrome (ARDS)
8. Circulatory collapse, shock, septicaemia (algid malaria)
9. Abnormal bleeding, jaundice, hemoglobinuria
10. High fever
11. Hyperparasitaemia (parasitaemia level of greater than 5%)

Table 11.2: Complications of severe malaria in pregnancy[3]

- Non-immune pregnant women → Risk of abortion, stillbirth, premature delivery, low infant birth weight, 2–10 times higher mortality from cerebral malaria, hypoglycemia, ARDS.
- Partially immune pregnant women → severe anemia.
- Maternal anemia—associated with maternal and perinatal morbidity and mortality
- Pulmonary oedema in anemic women after separation of placenta (if fluid overloaded or severely anemic)
- Fetal distress with poor prognosis
- Infections—pneumonia, urinary tract infection
- Hypoglycemia especially with quinine—sudden loss of consciousness, abnormal behavior, sweating, convulsions, decerebrate or decorticate rigidity

- Tissue sequestration of parasitized RBCs causes a more than expected severe fall in hemoglobin.

- Mortality >80%.
- May occur suddenly when patient is improving on treatment

Malaria with ARDS in Pregnancy: Worst Complication

- ARDS—increased pulmonary capillary permeability
- Tachypnoea, bilateral crepitations, reduced paO$_2$
- Hypoxia altered sensorium, death within hours
- Iatrogenic contribution fluid overload

Circulatory Collapse—Algid Malaria in Pregnancy

- Patient admitted in state of collapse with BP < 80 mmHg systolic, cold clammy skin, peripheral vasoconstriction, rapid thread pulse
- Predisposing factors—associated Gram negative septicaemia, metabolic acidosis, ARDS, massive GI hemorrhage, ruptured spleen

- Dehydration with hypovolemia contributory
- Search for infection (lungs, urinary and peripheral catheters, meninges)

Severe Malaria—Fluid and Electrolyte Disturbances in Pregnancy

- Hypovolaemia—low JVP/CVP, postural hypotension, oliguria with high urinary specific gravity, dry mucous membranes
- Acidotic breathing- hyperventilation, deep sighing 'Kussmaul's breathing'
- Lactic acidosis due to peripheral shock
- Hyperparasitaemia, hypoglycaemia, renal failure contributory

Malarial-Jaundice in Pregnancy

- High serum Bilirubin—indirect due to hemolysis, direct due to shock liver
- SGOT/SGPT: 3–5 fold elevation
- Hepatic encephalopathy with flaps
- Beware of hemolysis due to drugs in G6PD deficiency
- Excellent prognosis with standard treatment
- Mistaken for viral hepatitis.

Diagnosis

Peripheral smears of thick and thin blood films, thick for low density parasitaemia, thin for vivax/falciparum differentiation—remain the gold standard for diagnosis of malaria.[1]

Rapid diagnostic tests—stick or card tests using *Plasmodium falciparum* specific histidine—rich protein 2 or LDH antigens in finger prick blood samples are also available.

The poor prognostic indicators of severe malaria are listed in Table 11.3.[3,4]

Treatment

Quinine, chloroquine, clindamycin and proguanil are considered safe in 1st trimester. Artemisinin-based combination therapy (ACT) is considered safe in 2nd and 3rd trimesters.[1]

Treatment of Uncomplicated *P. Falciparum* Cases in Pregnancy

Artemisinin-based combination therapy (ACT)

1. Artemether (80 mg)—lumefantrine (480 mg) twice daily for 3 days
2. Artesunate 4 mg/kg body weight daily for 3 days + sulfadoxine (25 mg/kg body weight) + pyrimethamine (1.25 mg/kg body weight) on the first day.[1][e.g.: Tab malasulf (Sulfadoxine 500 plus pyrimethamine 25) 2 or 3 tablets stat]

Primaquine should be avoided in pregnant women.

Note: National Vector Borne Disease Control Programme (NVBDCP) (2013) recommends quinine salt 10 mg/kg 3 times daily for 7 days in **1st Trimester** and Artemisinin-based

Table 11.3: Poor prognostic indicators	
Clinical indicators	*Laboratory indicators*
1. Age under 3 years	1. Hyperparasitemia (>250 000/μl or >5%) peripheral schizontemia
2. Deep coma	2. Peripheral blood polymorphonuclear leucocytosis (>12 000/μl)
3. Witnessed or reported convulsions	3. Mature pigmented parasites (>20% parasites)
4. Decerebrate/decorticate rigidity or opisthotonous	4. WBCs with malaria pigment > 5%
5. Clinical signs of organ dysfunction (e.g. renal failure, pulmonary edema)	5. PCV <15% , Hb < 5g/dl, RBS <40 mg%
6. Respiratory distress (acidosis)	6. BUN> 60 mg/dl, creatinine > 3 mg/dl
7. Circulatory collapse	7. SGOT, SGPT > 120 IU/l, low AT III levels
8. Papilledema and /or retinal edema	8. High venous lactate > 5 mmol/l and CSF lactate > 6

combination therapy (ACT) in **2nd and 3rd trimester** for **uncomplicated** *P. falciparum* **cases.**[1]

Treatment of Severe and Complicated Malaria in Pregnancy[1,2]

1. Artesunate 2.4 mg/kg loading dose IV or IM followed by 1.2 mg/kg @ 12 and 24 hrs; and daily for 7 days.
2. Artemether 3.2 mg/kg loading dose IM followed by 1.6 mg/kg/day × 7 days.
3. Caution: Artesunate and Artemether are soluble only at an alkaline pH; hence should be reconstituted only in 5% soda bicarbonate solution (provided with the drug ampoule) (It precipitates in saline/ glucose)

Severe Malaria in Pregnancy General Management[2,3]

- Hematological and biochemical investigations, ECG, X-ray Chest, ABG
- MICU admission, monitor RBS, vital parameters monitoring, RT, Foleys, cavafix/ central line insertion
- Monitor urine output, core temperature, respiratory rate
- Blood cultures if shock. Antibiotics– ceftriaxone + metronidazole.
- Avoid corticosteroids, aspirin
- Convulsions—Diazepam 0.15 mg/kg slow IV or IM, or paraaldehyde 0.1 mg/kg
- Fresh blood/packed cells with sos IV Furosemide 20 mg for circulatory overload
- 25% glucose 100 cc IV 6 hrly.
- Tepid sponging, paracetamol

In addition, the various complications of severe malaria listed above should be treated symptomatically, e.g. haemodialysis for renal failure, ventilator with IPPV and PEEP for ARDS.

Note: Pregnant women with severe malaria in any trimester can be treated with artemisinin derivatives, which in contrast to quinine, do not risk aggravating hypo-glycemia.

DENGUE

Dengue is a disease caused by virus serotypes of the genus Flavivirus, family flaviviridae. It is spread by Aedes aegypti mosquito. Commonly seen in children but with increasing rate of adult infection, the number of infected pregnant women has also increased.[5]

Clinical Features

Classic dengue fever: It is characterised by fever, headache, retro-orbital pain, myalgia, classically described as break bone fever. Fever with rigors up to 105–106°F, leukopenia, thrombocytopenia are common manifestations. It resolves in 5–6 days.[6]

This classic fever can also take a complicated course leading to dengue shock syndrome and dengue hemorrhagic fever.

The WHO criteria for DSS (Dengue Shock Syndrome)[7] are given in Table 11.4.

The WHO criteria for DHF (Dengue Hemorrhagic Fever)[7] are given in Table 11.5.

Table 11.4: WHO criteria for DSS (dengue shock syndrome)[7]

1. Rapid weak pulse
2. Pulse pressure ≤ 20 mmHg
3. Hypotension with cold clammy extremities
4. Restlessness

Table 11.5: WHO criteria for DHF (dengue hemorrhagic fever)[7]

- Fever—acute onset, continuous for 2–7 days
- Hemorrhagic manifestation—positive tourniquet test PLUS any one of—petechiae, purpura, ecchymosis, epistaxis, bleeding gums, hematemesis/malena.
- Thrombocytopenia ≤ 1,00,000/cumm
- Plasma leakage evidenced by at least one of the following:
  a. Rise in hematocrit > 20%
  b. Pleural effusion, ascitis, hypoalbuminea

Diagnosis

The diagnosis of dengue fever may be confirmed by microbiological laboratory testing. This can be done by viral antigen detection (such as for NS1) or specific antibodies (serology), virus isolation in cell cultures, nucleic acid detection by PCR. Detection of NS1 during the febrile phase of a primary infection may be > 90% sensitive. Tests for dengue virus-specific antibodies, types IgG and IgM, can be useful in confirming a diagnosis in the later stages of the infection. Both IgG and IgM are produced after 5–7 days. The highest levels (titres) of IgM are detected following a primary infection, but IgM is also produced in re-infection with a different serovar. IgG antibodies are non-specific as it can be present in old infection.[5,6]

Treatment

No drug or vaccine is available for the treatment of dengue/DHF. The control of Aedes Aegypti mosquito is the only method of choice. Early detection with proper case management and symptomatic treatment can reduce mortality substantially. Management of dengue fever is mainly symptomatic and supportive.[5, 6]

In DHF/DSS, the following treatment is recommended:[6–8]

- Correct circulatory collapse with ½ normal dextrose saline 40 ml/kg to restore BP, then slow to 10 ml/kg/hr. Plasma expanders—colloids (haemaccel) may be needed.
- Nasal O_2 with high flow mask
- Rx of shock—CVP line/IV fluids, inotropes
- Frank DIC—fresh frozen plasma 2–4 units/day till FDP and Sr. fibrinogen stabilize; platelet transfusion 2–4 units at time if platelet count < 20,000/cumm.
- PCV transfusion for massive GI hemorrhage
- IV Methyl prednisolone 125 mg × 3–5 days
- Ventilator with IPPV and PEEP for ARDS
- Salicylates and sympathomimetic amines are contraindicated.

LEPTOSPIROSIS

Leptospirosis is a direct zoonotic disease caused by spirochetes belonging to the genus Leptospira. Human infection results from accidental contact with carrier animals or environment contaminated with animal urine containing the organism. The majority of leptospiral infections are either subclinical or result in very mild illness and patients recover without complications. In a few cases it may manifest as multiorgan failure with a mortality of up to 40%.[9]

Infection in pregnant women may be grave leading to severe fetal and maternal morbidity and mortality. The presentation may mimic acute fatty liver, pregnancy induced hypertension, and HELLP syndrome. Owing to the unusual presentation, leptospirosis in pregnancy is often misdiagnosed and under-reported.[9]

Clinical Features

Leptospirosis can manifest in many ways. The various syndromes of presentation are as follows:

1. Anicteric leptospirosis
2. Icteric leptospirosis (Weil's disease)
3. Hemorrhagic fever with renal syndrome
4. Atypical pneumonia syndrome hemorrhagic ARDS
5. Myocarditis
6. Aseptic meningoencephalitis
7. Ocular manifestations

The incubation period is 7–14 days, but ranges from 2–21 days. 90% or more of all cases of leptospirosis are anicteric. In general both anicteric and icteric cases follow a biphasic course 'septicaemia' or 'leptospiremic' phase.[10]

Anicteric Leptospirosis

This can be mild with fever, headache, and body pains or more severe when it is a biphasic illness. The onset is abrupt with chills, rigor, fever (temperature 30–40°C), nausea and vomiting, severe headache and body pain. The body aches are severe and most marked in the lower limbs especially thighs and calves. Chest pain, dry cough and hemoptysis may occur. Mental symptoms such as restlessness, confusion, delirium, and occasional psychotic behavior may occur. The most characteristic findings on examination are conjunctival suffusion and severe myalgia. The 'septicaemia' phase subsides after 4–7 days. The second or immune phase is characterized by severe headache due to meningeal involvement, uveitis and low grade fever. This lasts from 4 to 30 days longer. The biphasic course may not be seen in all patients.[10]

Icteric Leptospirosis (Weil's disease)

In some patients, the septicemic phase instead of subsiding, progresses to a severe icteric illness with renal failure. Meningeal symptoms are frequent, but are overshadowed by hepatic or renal features. Severe bleeding, hypotension, cardiac and pulmonary complications are frequent. Death occurs usually due to renal failure. Sudden death may occur due to massive bleeding, arrhythmias or cardiac and respiratory failure. In those who are not severely ill, diuresis occurs and renal failure improves. The fever subsides and the general condition gradually improves.[10]

Diagnosis[11,12]

ELISA: It detects genus-specific IgM antibodies for rapid diagnosis of current infection.

Culture: The isolation of leptospirosis by culture of blood, CSF and urine is the most definite way of confirming the diagnosis of leptospirosis.

PCR is promising on both sensitivity and specificity, but is complicated and expensive. (Modified Faine's Criteria (with Amendment) 2012 is used for diagnosis of leptospirosis)[12]

Treatment

Penicillin is the most effective antibiotic when given early. In severe illness large doses (1.5 million units every 6 hourly) of benzyl penicillin may be given, preferably by IV route, for 10–14 days. Fever subsides in 24–36 hours. In resistant cases, cefotaxime (1 g IV q6h) and ceftriaxone (1 g IV BD) for 10–14 days are effective against leptospira. Doxycycline and quinolones should be avoided in pregnancy.[10]

Symptomatic and supportive treatment: Of primary importance is the meticulous attention to fluid and electrolyte balance. Hypovolaemia and hypotension need prompt and specific treatment with intravenous fluids. In patient with oliguria, if pre-renal azotaemia is suspected, prompt diuresis should be attempted with fluid therapy. Patients who have no response to therapy should be managed as established renal failure. Headache and myalgia are treated with analgesics; fever with antipyretics, restlessness and anxiety with sedatives and anemia with blood transfusion. IV methyl prednisolone (250–500 mg) for 3 days can be given for ARDS.[10]

HEPATITIS E

Hepatitis E is caused by the hepatitis E virus (HEV). The incubation period ranges from three to eight weeks, with a mean of 40 days. The period of communicability is unknown. Pica of pregnancy increases the urge to have roadside food which possesses a grave danger for hepatitis E infection.[13]

Pregnancy appears to be a potential risk factor for viral replication. It has been reported that a significant proportion of pregnant women with acute hepatitis E progress to acute liver failure with a short pre-encephalo-pathy period, rapid development of cerebral edema and high occurrence of disseminated intravascular coagulation. This is attributed to the high level of steroid hormones, in pregnancy, which are immunosuppressive.

These steroid hormones may also promote viral replication. It has a direct inhibition on hepatic cells, which may predispose to hepatic dysfunction/failure when exposed to infectious pathogens.[13]

Clinical Features

Typical signs and symptoms of hepatitis include:

- Fever
- Jaundice (yellow discolouration of the skin and sclera of the eyes, dark urine and pale stools)
- Anorexia (loss of appetite)
- Nausea and vomiting
- Abdominal pain and tenderness
- An enlarged, tender liver (hepatomegaly).

Diagnosis[14]

Diagnosis of hepatitis E infection is based on the detection of specific IgM antibodies to the virus in the blood. Additional tests include reverse transcriptase polymerase chain reaction (RT-PCR) to detect the hepatitis E virus RNA in blood and/or stool.

Complications

During pregnancy, the risk of fulminant HEV disease is high and maternal mortality occurs in 20% when the disease presents in third trimester. Premature deliveries with high infant mortality of up to 33% are also observed. Although the mechanism underlying the increased mortality is unknown, the reported complications include gestational hypertension, preeclampsia, proteinuria, edema, and kidney disease. The most severe complication is acute liver failure leading to cerebral edema and hepatic encephalopathy.[13,14]

Treatment

There is no available treatment capable of altering the course of acute hepatitis. Prevention is the most effective approach against the disease. Therapy is directed at providing supportive care and treating the complications preferably in the setting of a medical intensive care unit. Treatment of acute liver failure leading to cerebral edema and hepatic encephalopathy is as follows.[15]

Grade I/II Encephalopathy

1. *CT brain:* To rule out other causes of decreased mental status; little a utility to identify cerebral edema
2. Avoid stimulation and sedate if possible
3. *Antibiotics:* Surveillance and treatment of infection required; prophylaxis possibly helpful
4. Lactulose (oral or rectal), possibly helpful
5. Injection vitamin K and Fresh Frozen Plasma for coagulation abnormalities.
6. Consider transfer to liver transplant facility and listing for transplantation.

Grade III/IV Encephalopathy

1. Intubate the patient (may require sedation)
2. Elevate head end of bed
3. Consider placement of ICP monitoring device
4. Immediate treatment of seizures required (if any); prophylaxis of unclear value
5. Mannitol (0.5–1.0 gm/kg body weight OD or BD): used if ICP severely elevated or first clinical signs of herniation.
6. Hypertonic saline (3% NACL) to raise serum sodium to 145–155 mmol/L (used in severe cases like serum ammonia >150 µM, grade 3/4 hepatic encephalopathy, acute renal failure, requiring vasopressors to maintain MAP)
7. *Hyperventilation:* Effects short-lived; may use for impending herniation

TYPHOID

Typhoid and paratyphoid fevers are commonly grouped together under the collective term 'enteric fever'. Typhoid is caused by *Salmonella typhi* and paratyphoid is caused by either *Salmonella paratyphi* A, B, or C. Typhoid and paratyphoid are transmitted mainly by the faecal-oral route through unhygienic food and water.[16]

Clinical Features[16]

- Typhoid patients often have continuous fevers that run as high as 103 or 104°F (39 to 40°C).
- Headaches
- Poor appetite
- Generalized aches and pains
- Lethargy, weakness, and fatigue
- Diarrhoea
- Rash (rose-colored sports on the lower chest and upper abdomen).

If untreated, a second stage of typhoid may result with a continuation of a high fever, severe constipation or diarrhea that resembles pea soup, extreme weight loss, and an uncomfortable, distended abdomen.

The final stage of symptoms leaves a person delirious with variable degrees of unconsciousness in later stages. On treatment a slow improvement is seen with gradual defervescence of the fever.

Diagnosis[16,17]

A number of serologic tests, including the classic Widal test, are available to detect *S. typhi* antigen or antibody. But definitive diagnosis of enteric fever requires the isolation of *S. typhi* or *S. paratyphi*. Cultures of blood, stool, urine and bone marrow may each be useful in establishing the diagnosis. The sensitivity of blood culture alone is 50 to 70%. The sensitivity of bone marrow culture is 90% and, unlike blood culture, is not influenced by up to 5 days of prior antimicrobial therapy.

Treatment

There are a few data on the treatment of typhoid in pregnancy. The beta-lactams are considered safe. Fluoroquinolones are not recommended in pregnancy.

Intravenous ceftriaxone, 50–75 mg/kg/day (2–4 g per day) in one or two doses for seven days can be used in pregnant women. Another regime is azithromycin in a dose of 500 mg (10 mg/kg) given once daily for seven days. In resistant cases piperacillin-tazobactam 4.5 gm IV 8 hrly can be used. Treatment duration may need to be extended to 14 days depending on the clinical response.[16,17]

SWINE FLU

It is a human respiratory infection caused by H1N1 strain of influenza virus, popularly known as swine flu. It was first recognized in spring 2009 after which the World Health Organization declared the infection a global pandemic in August 2010.

Note: The H1N1 viral strain implicated in the 2009 flu pandemic was earlier referred to as "swine flu" because initial testing showed that many of the genes in the virus were similar to influenza viruses which were normally occurring in North American swine. But further research has shown that the outbreak is due to a reassortant strains of H1N1 not previously reported in pigs.[18]

About the virus: It is an enveloped RNA virus, 80–200 nm, of the family orthomyxoviridae. The virus contains two surface antigens H (hemagluttinin) and N (neuraminidase). It is transmitted through droplet infection.[18]

Incubation period: Not specified but can range from one to seven days.[18]

Clinical Manifestations

The clinical presentation of the H1N1 influenza is fever, cough, sore throat, malaise, headache; vomiting and diarrhea. Pregnant women form the high risk group along with children, elderly and immunodeficient patients. Pregnant women can present with the above symptoms followed by breathlessness with features suggestive of acute lung injury (ALI) including hypoxia which can relentlessly progress to full blown acute respiratory distress syndrome (ARDS) within hours with high fatality rates. Suspicion is high if there is a history of close contact within 7 days with a probable or confirmed case of the influenza (H1N1) virus infection **OR** travel history within 7 days to a place with one or more confirmed influenza (H1N1) cases.[18]

Diagnosis[19]

Various diagnostic tools are used for detection of H1N1 virus. The commonly used ones include:

- *RT-PCR:* It is the method of choice for diagnosing H1N1 as per CDC. The Human Influenza Virus Real-Time RT-PCR Detection and Characterization Panel (RT-PCR Flu Panel) can provide results within 4 hours. It is the only *in vitro* diagnostic test for influenza that is cleared by the FDA for use with lower respiratory tract specimens.
- Rapid influenza diagnostic tests (RIDTs) and direct Immunofluorescence Assays (DFAs) are widely available but have variable sensitivity for detecting H1N1 influenza when compared with RT-PCR.
- Viral culture
- Four-fold rise in new influenza A (H1N1) virus-specific neutralizing antibodies.

Treatment

Laboratory confirmation of influenza virus infection is not necessary for the initiation of treatment and a negative laboratory test for H1N1 does not exclude the diagnosis in all patients. Early empirical treatment with Oseltamivir 75 mg BD for 5 days is strongly recommended in pregnant women with typical signs and symptoms or with history of contacts with H1N1 cases. Higher doses of Oseltamivir (150 mg) and longer duration of treatment may be appropriate in critical cases, although there is no available clinical trial evidence. Dose adjustment is needed in renal impairment.[18,20]

Antiviral resistance: Zanamivir is the treatment of choice for all patients where oseltamivir resistance is demonstrated or highly suspected. Intravenous zanamivir may be considered if available.[18,20]

Prevention of Monsoon Fevers in Pregnancy

Almost all monsoons related illnesses are communicable diseases. These dangerous diseases can be prevented by using simple methods of maintaining personal hygiene and good sanitation through public education, mass media and law enforcing agencies.

REFERENCES

1. www.nvbdcp.gov.in/Doc/Diagnosis-Treatment-Malaria-2013 (Last accessed: 20/5/15)
2. Malaria in Pregnancy-Hiralal Konar, Picklu Chaudhari (Treatment and prognosis in obstetrics and gynecology, Page 126)
3. Guidelines for the Treatment of Malaria. 2nd ed. Geneva: World Health Organization; 2010 (www.who.int/malaria/publications/atoz/9789241547925/en/index.html).(Last accessed: 15/5/15)
4. Royal College of Obstetricians and Gynaecologists (RCOG)—The diagnosis and treatment of malaria in pregnancy, April 2010 London (UK).(www.rcog.org.uk)(Last accessed—20/5/15)
5. Dengue Guidelines For Diagnosis,Treatment, Prevention and Control, 2009. (http://www.who.int/tdr/publications/documents/dengue-diagnosis.pdf) (Last accessed: 20/5/15)
6. WHO. Dengue and dengue haemorrhagic fever. Factsheet No 117, revised May 2008. Geneva, World Health Organization, 2008 (http://www.who.int/mediacentre/ factsheets/fs117/en/). (Last accessed: 1/6/15)
7. Dengue Hemorrhagic Fever and Dengue Shock Syndrome —Pertinent Issues in Management-Sk Sharma, Ashish Goel (www.apiindia.org/pdf/medicine_update_2007/107.pdf) (Last accessed: 2/6/15)
8. Clinical Practice Guidelines on Management of Dengue Infection in Adults (Revised 2nd Edition) 2010. (http://www.moh.gov.my/attachments/5502.pdf)

9. Leptospirosis in pregnancy-Puliyath G, Singh S.(http://www.ncbi.nlm.nih.gov/pubmed/22549729) (Last accessed: 2/6/15).

10. Approach to leptospirosis in India- S.Shivakumar (http://www.drshivakumar.org) (Last accessed: 2/6/15)

11. Human leptospirosis : Guidance for diagnosis, surveillance and control (http://www.who.int/csr/don/en/WHO_CDS_CSR_EPH_2002.23.pdf) (Last accessed: 18/5/15)

12. Faine S. guidelines for the control of Leptospirosis. WHO offset publication.1982; 67.

13. Hepatitis E Virus Infection DuringPregnancy: Why Is The Disease Stormy? PremashisKar, New Delhi (http://www.apiindia.org/pdf/medicine_update_2012/hepatology_02.pdf).

14. Aggarwal R, Krawczynski K. Hepatitis E: An overview and recent advances in clinical and laboratory research. J Gastroenterol Hepatol 2000; 15:9–20.

15. AASLD Position Paper: The Management of Acute Liver Failure: Update 2011-William M. Lee, Anne M. Larson, R. Todd Stravitz.

16. Management of Enteric Fever In 2012 Falguni S. Parikh (http://www.apiindia.org/pdf/medicine_update_2012/infectious_disease_03.pdf)(Last accessed: 5/6/15)

17. The diagnosis, treatment and prevention of typhoid fever (www.who.int/rpc/TFGuideWHO) (Last accessed: 25/5/15)

18. Pandemic Influenza (H1N1) 2009: Monthly Newsletter of National Centre for Disease Control, Directorate General of Health Services, Government of India(http://www.ncdc.gov.in/writereaddata/linkimages/Aug-Sep_092813460594.pdf) (Last accessed: 5/6/15)

19. H1N1 Flu: Diagnosis and Lab Testing-Centres for disease control and prevention (http://www.cdc.gov/h1n1flu/diagnostic_testing_clinicians_qa.htm) (Last accessed: 5/6/15)

20. WHO Guidelines for Pharmacological Management of Pandemic Influenza A(H1N1) 2009 and other Influenza Viruses (http://www.who.int/csr/resources/publications/swineflu/h1n1_guidelines_pharmaceutical_mngt.pdf) (Last accessed: 5/6/15)

Section

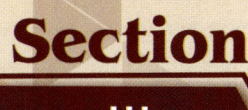

III

Specific Situations

12

Urinary Tract Infections in Pregnancy

Neelam N Redkar, Prakash Ram Relwani

INTRODUCTION

Urinary tract infections (UTI) are one of the most common infections in pregnancy.[1] Due to several anatomical and hormonal changes, pregnant women are more susceptible to urinary tract infections.[2] Prevalence of symptomatic and asymptomatic bacteriuria was found to be 19.87% and 4.34% respectively in an Indian study done by Bandyopadhyay S et al.[3]

Asymptomatic bacteriuria associated with pregnancy has a direct bearing not only on the health of the women but also on pregnancy and hence needs to be diagnosed and treated appropriately. Asymptomatic bacteriuria can lead to cystitis and pyelonephritis.

UTI is more common in females as factors like short urethra and easy contamination of the urinary tract with fecal contamination makes them susceptible. In pregnancy additional factors like increased bladder volume with decreased tone causes urinary stasis.

If untreated, UTI during pregnancy causes complications like acute pyelonephritis, anemia, sepsis, renal failure and shock and fetal complications like intrauterine growth restriction (IUGR), acute respiratory distress syndrome and prematurity.

DEFINITION

Urinary tract infection: UTI is defined as the presence of at least 10^5 organisms per milliliter of urine in an asymptomatic patient, or as more than 100 organisms/mL of urine with accompanying pyuria (> 7 white blood cells [WBCs]/mL) in a symptomatic patient.

ETIOLOGY

E. coli is the most common cause of UTI, accounting for approximately 60–80% of cases.[4,5] It originates from fecal flora colonizing the periurethral area, causing an ascending infection. Other pathogens include the following:[6]

- *Klebsiella pneumoniae*
- Proteus mirabilis
- Enterobacter species
- *Staphylococcus saprophyticus*
- Group B beta-hemolytic Streptococcus (GBS)

Infection with *S. saprophyticus*, an aggressive community-acquired organism, can cause upper urinary tract disease, and this infection is more likely to be persistent or recurrent.

Urea-splitting bacteria, including Proteus, Klebsiella, Pseudomonas, and coagulase-negative Staphylococcus, alkalinize the urine and may be associated with struvite stones. Chlamydial infections are associated with sterile pyuria and account for more than 30% of atypical pathogens.

GBS colonization has important implications during pregnancy. Intrapartum transmission that leads to neonatal GBS infection can cause pneumonia, meningitis, sepsis, and death.

PATHOPHYSIOLOGY

Infections result from ascending colonization of the urinary tract, primarily by existing vaginal, perineal, and fecal flora. Various maternal physiologic and anatomic factors predispose to ascending infection. Such factors include urinary retention caused by the weight of the enlarging uterus and urinary stasis due to progesterone-induced ureteral smooth muscle relaxation. Blood-volume expansion is accompanied by increases in the glomerular filtration rate and urinary output.

Loss of ureteral tone combined with increased urinary tract volume results in urinary stasis, which can lead to dilatation of the ureters, renal pelvis, and calyces.

Calyceal and ureteral dilatation are more common on the right side; in 86% of cases, the dilatation is localized to the right and also the dilatation is more pronounced on the right than the left (average 15 mm vs 5 mm). This dilatation appears to begin by about 10 weeks' gestation and worsens throughout pregnancy. This is underscored by the distribution of cases of pyelonephritis during pregnancy: 2% during the first trimester, 52% during the second trimester, and 46% in the third trimester.

Glycosuria and an increase in levels of urinary amino acids (aminoaciduria) during pregnancy are additional factors that lead to UTI.

CLINICAL PRESENTATION

Asymptomatic Bacteriuria

Asymptomatic bacteriuria is commonly defined as the presence of more than 10^5 organisms/mL in 2 consecutive urine samples in the absence of symptoms. Untreated asymptomatic bacteriuria leads to the development of symptomatic cystitis in approximately 30 percent of patients and can lead to the development of pyelonephritis in up to 50 percent.[7] Asymptomatic bacteriuria has been associated with low birthweight and preterm delivery.[8]

Symptomatic Bacteriuria

It is classified into lower tract infection and upper tract infections, according to the anatomical site of contamination

- *Lower UTIs:* The anatomical site of the infection can be the bladder (cystitis) and/or the urethra (urethritis)
- *Upper UTIs:* The kidneys are the anatomical site of the infection (pyelonephritis associated with inflammation of the renal parenchyma, calices and pelvis)

Acute Cystitis

Acute cystitis involves only the lower urinary tract; it is characterized by inflammation of the bladder. Signs and symptoms include dysuria, suprapubic discomfort, frequency, urgency, and nocturia. These symptoms are often difficult to distinguish from those due to pregnancy itself.

Acute Pyelonephritis

Pyelonephritis is the most common complication of UTI in pregnant women. Acute pyelonephritis is characterized by fever, flank pain, and tenderness in addition to significant bacteriuria. Other symptoms may include nausea, vomiting, frequency, urgency, and dysuria. Furthermore, women with additional risk factors (e.g. immunosuppression, diabetes, sickle cell anemia, neurogenic bladder, recurrent or persistent UTIs before pregnancy) are at an increased risk for a complicated UTI.

Complications

Maternal
- Acute pyelonephritis
- Perinephric cellulitis and abscess
- Septic shock
- Acute kidney injury
- Acute lung injury

Fetal

- Hypoxic fetal events due to maternal complications of infection that lead to hypoperfusion of the placenta.
- Premature delivery leading to increased infant morbidity and mortality.

Schieve and associates [9] conducted a study involving 25,746 pregnant women and found that the presence of UTI was associated with premature labor (labor onset before 37 weeks of gestation), hypertensive disorders of pregnancy (such as pregnancy-induced hypertension and preeclampsia), anemia (hematocrit level less than 30 percent) and amnionitis.

The development of preeclampsia is associated with maternal UTI (asymptomatic bacteriuria or symptomatic infection) during pregnancy.[8]

SCREENING

The American Congress of Obstetrics and Gynecology recommends that a urine culture should be obtained at the first prenatal visit.[10] A repeat urine culture should be obtained during the third trimester, because the urine of treated patients may not remain sterile for the entire pregnancy.[10] The recommendation of the US Preventive Services Task Force is to obtain a urine culture between 12 and 16 weeks of gestation.[11]

By screening for and aggressively treating pregnant women with asymptomatic bacteriuria, it is possible to significantly decrease the annual incidence of pyelonephritis during pregnancy.[12,13] In randomized controlled trials, treatment of pregnant women with asymptomatic bacteriuria has been shown to decrease the incidence of preterm birth and low-birth-weight infants.[14]

Rouse and colleagues[15] performed a cost-benefit analysis of screening for bacteriuria in pregnant women versus inpatient treatment of pyelonephritis and found a substantial decrease in overall cost with screening.

The accuracy of faster screening methods (e.g. leukocyte esterase dipstick, nitrite dipstick, urinalysis and urine Gram staining) has been evaluated. Bachman and associates[16] compared these screening methods with urine culture and found that although it was more cost effective to screen for bacteriuria with the esterase dipstick for leukocytes, but the increased number of false negatives and the relatively poor predictive value of a positive test make the faster methods less useful; therefore, a urine culture should be routinely obtained in pregnant women to screen for bacteriuria at the first prenatal visit and during the third trimester.[9,10]

Urine Studies

In all pregnant patients, a urine specimen should be carefully collected for urinalysis and culturing during the first prenatal visit or at 12–16 weeks' gestation. These tests help to identify patients with asymptomatic bacteriuria, as well as those with other concerning findings such as glycosuria.

For urine collection, a midstream clean catch is adequate.

Urine Culture

Urine culture is the standard method for evaluating for urinary tract infection (UTI) during pregnancy. Urine culture is absolutely indicated in the following conditions:

- Pyelonephritis
- Failure to respond to initial treatment regimens
- History of recent instrumentation
- Hospital admission

Two consecutive voided specimens with isolation of the same bacterial strain, at a colony count of 10^5 colony-forming units (CFUs) per milliliter or higher, has historically been used to define a positive culture result. A single catheterized specimen yielding a colony count of at least 100 CFU/mL is also diagnostic. Counts lower than 10^5 CFU/mL, with 2 or more organisms, usually indicate specimen contamination rather than infection.

Culture results can be used to identify specific organisms and antibiotic sensitivities.

Blood Studies

The following blood tests should be ordered at the physician's discretion:

- Complete blood count (CBC)
- Serum electrolytes
- Blood urea nitrogen (BUN)
- Serum creatinine

Renal Ultrasonography and Intravenous Pyelography

Unless an anatomic abnormality or renal disease is suspected, initial routine imaging studies are not necessary. Patients with suspected pyelonephritis who are not responsive to appropriate antibiotic therapy after 48–72 hours should also undergo imaging.

The total dosage of ionizing radiation should not exceed 3–5 cGy during the course of pregnancy. A limited IVP can deliver 0.4–1 cGy radiation.

Treatment

Pregnant women should be treated when bacteriuria is identified. The choice of antibiotic should address the most common infecting organisms (i.e. gram-negative gastrointestinal organisms).The antibiotic should also be safe for the mother and fetus.

As per an Indian study done by Mathai et al[17] about 90% of E. coli causing UTI is still susceptible to nitrofurantoin, a relatively inexpensive and safe drug. There was high prevalence of resistance to amoxycillin.

Historically, ampicillin has been the drug of choice, but in recent years E. coli has become increasingly resistant to ampicillin.[18] Ampicillin resistance is found in 20 to 30 percent of E. coli cultured from urine in the outpatient setting.[19]

Some antibiotics should not be used during pregnancy, because of their effects on the fetus.

Antibiotic	Category	Effect on fetus
Tetracyclines	D	Adverse effect on fetal teeth and bones
Trimethoprim	C	Facial defects and the first trimester cardiac abnormalities
Sulfonamides in the third trimester	C	Jaundice and kernicterus
Chloramphenicol	C	Gray syndrome
Fluoroquinolones	C	Cartilage defects

Data are insufficient to recommend any specific regimen.[20,21] The following strategies are based on evaluation of review articles.[10,22]

ASYMPTOMATIC BACTERIURIA AND ACUTE CYSTITIS

Nitrofurantoin is generally considered first-line treatment. Nitrofurantoin has high concentrations in the urinary tract but induces minimal resistance in gram-negative organisms. If nitrofurantoin is not effective, change antibiotics based on urine culture antibiotic sensitivity profiles. Single-dose treatment for pregnant women with asymptomatic bacteriuria has been evaluated, given its lower cost and better compliance. However, evidence is insufficient to determine whether single-dose or longer-duration regimens are more effective.[23] 7–10 days of treatment is usually recommended to eradicate the offending bacteria. Treatment success depends on eradication of the bacteria rather than on the duration of therapy. A test-for-cure urine culture should show negative findings 1–2 weeks after therapy. Antibiotics commonly used are:

First-line therapy
Nitrofurantoin 100 mg orally twice daily
Amoxicillin 500 mg orally twice daily
Amoxicillin-clavulanate 500/125 mg orally twice daily
Cephalexin 500 mg orally twice daily
Cefuroxime 250 mg orally twice daily

Second-line therapy
Fosfomycin 3 g orally as single dose
Duration of therapy is 7–10 days

PYELONEPHRITIS

The standard course of treatment for pyelonephritis consists of hospital admission and intravenous (IV) administration of beta lactams with or without aminoglycosides (Category D) for 10–14 days.[24] The decision regarding antibiotics should be based on culture. Patients with pyelonephritis can become dehydrated because of nausea and vomiting and need IV hydration.

Antibiotic	Dose
Ceftriaxone	1–2 gm every 24 hr single dose or in 2 divided doses
Cefotaxime	1–2 gm every 8 hr
Piperacillin-tazobactam	4.5 gm every 8 hr
Meropenem	500 mg every 8 hr
Imipenem-Cilastatin	500 mg every 6 hr

In a randomized, controlled trial of outpatient treatment of pyelonephritis in pregnancy, Millar et al concluded that outpatient therapy is as safe and effective as inpatient care in the treatment of pyelonephritis before 24 weeks'gestation.[25] Pyelonephritis places the patient at risk for spontaneous abortion in early pregnancy and for preterm labor after 24 weeks' gestation. If outpatient therapy is considered, only selected patients in their second trimester should be considered. More study is necessary before a change in the above practice pattern is considered. However, the prevailing view is still that aggressive inpatient hydration and parenteral antibiotics are necessary.

SPECIAL CONSIDERATIONS

Group B Streptococcal Infection

Group B streptococcal (GBS) vaginal colonization is known to be a cause of neonatal sepsis and is associated with preterm rupture of membranes, and preterm labor and delivery. GBS is found to be the causative organism in UTIs in approximately 5 percent of patients.[26,27] Current recommendations are that women with documented group B streptococcal bacteriuria (regardless of level of colony-forming units per mL) in the current pregnancy should be treated at the time of labor or rupture of membranes with appropriate intravenous antibiotics for the prevention of early-onset neonatal group B streptococcal disease.[28] Prophylaxis (usually with penicillin G) is given during labor. It is unclear if GBS bacteriuria is equivalent to GBS vaginal colonization, but pregnant women with GBS bacteriuria should be treated as GBS carriers and should receive a prophylactic antibiotic during labor.

Surgical Treatment

In patients with urethral or bladder diverticulum, bladder stones, lower urinary tract trauma, interstitial cystitis, or bladder cancer, cystoscopy may aid in establishing the diagnosis.

A retrograde stent or a percutaneous nephrostomy tube should be placed to relieve ureteral colic or decompress an obstructed infected collecting system. More invasive procedures, such as ureteroscopic stone extraction, are rarely indicated. Extracorporeal shock wave lithotripsy (ESWL) is contraindicated in pregnancy.

In the rare patient for whom invasive surgical therapy is indicated, the operation should be planned for the second trimester. Surgical intervention during the first trimester is associated with miscarriage; surgery in the third trimester is associated with preterm labor. Urgent surgical intervention in the third trimester should coincide with delivery of the fetus.

RECURRENCE AND PROPHYLAXIS

The majority of UTIs are caused by gastrointestinal organisms. Even with appropriate treatment, the patient may experience a reinfection of the urinary tract from the rectal reservoir. UTIs recur in approximately 4 to 5 percent of pregnancies, and the risk of developing pyelonephritis is the same as the risk with primary UTIs. A single, postcoital dose or daily suppression with cephalexin (125–250 mg) or nitrofurantoin (50–100 mg) in patients with recurrent UTIs is effective preventive therapy except during the last 4 weeks of pregnancy.[29] A postpartum urologic evaluation may be necessary in patients with recurrent infections because they are more likely to have structural abnormalities of the renal system. Patients who are found to have urinary stones, who have more than one recurrent UTI or who have a recurrent UTI while on suppressive antibiotic therapy should undergo a postpartum evaluation.

SUMMARY

UTIs are common during pregnancy, and the most common causative organism is *E. Coli.* UTIs during pregnancy are a common cause of serious maternal and perinatal morbidity. With appropriate screening and treatment, this morbidity can be limited. A UTI may manifest as asymptomatic bacteriuria, acute cystitis or pyelonephritis. Asymptomatic bacteriuria can lead to the development of cystitis or pyelonephritis. All pregnant women should be screened for asymptomatic bacteriuria and subsequently treated with antibiotics. Acute cystitis and pyelonephritis should be aggressively treated during pregnancy. Oral nitrofurantoin is a good antibiotic choice for treatment in pregnant women with asymptomatic bacteriuria and acute cystitis, but parenteral antibiotic therapy is required in women with pyelonephritis.

REFERENCES

1. Mittal P, Wing DA, Urinary tract infections in pregnancy, ClinPerinatol. 2005 Sep;32(3):749–64.
2. Dafnis E, Sabatini S, The effect of pregnancy on renal function: physiology and pathophysiology, Am J Med Sci 1992, 303(3):184–205.
3. High prevalence of bacteriuria in pregnancy and its screening methods in north India, Bandyopadhyay S, Thakur JS, Ray P, Kumar R, Journal of the Indian Medical Association [2005, 103(5):259–62, 266].
4. Hooton TM. Pathogenesis of urinary tract infections: an update. J Antimicrob Chemother. 2000;46(Suppl A):1–7.
5. KS Saraswathi, Farhana Aljabri, Incidence of urinary tract infections in pregnant women of tertiary care hospital, Der Pharmacia Lettre, 2013, 5(1):265–268.
6. Nicolle LE, Bradley S, Colgan R, Rice JC, Schaeffer A, Hooton TM. Infectious Diseases Society of America guidelines for the diagnosis and treatment of asymptomatic bacteriuria in adults. Clin Infect Dis. Mar 1 2005;40(5):643–54.
7. Kass EH. Pregnancy, pyelonephritis and prematurity. ClinObstet Gynecol. 1970;13:239–54.
8. Minassian C, Thomas SL, Williams DJ, Campbell O, Smeeth L. Acute maternal infection and risk of pre-eclampsia: A population-based case-control study. PLoS One. Sep 3 2013;8(9):e73047.
9. Schieve LA, Handler A, Hershow R, Persky V, Davis F. Urinary tract infection during pregnancy: Its association with maternal morbidity and perinatal outcome. Am J Public Health. 1994; 84:405–10.
10. Antimicrobial therapy for obstetric patients. ACOG educational bulletin no. 245. Washington, DC: American College of Obstetricians and Gynecologists, March 1998;245:8–10.
11. US Preventive Services Task Force. Guide to clinical preventive services: report of the US Preventive Services Task Force. 2d ed. Baltimore: Williams & Wilkins, 1996.
12. Gratacos E, Torres PJ, Vila J, Alonso PL, Cararach V. Screening and treatment of asymptomatic bacteriuria in pregnancy prevent pyelonephritis. J Infect Dis. 1994;169:1390–2.
13. Harris RE. The significance of eradication of bacteriuria during pregnancy.Obstet Gynecol. 1979;53:71–3.
14. Romero R, Oyarzun E, Mazor M, Sirtori M, Hobbins JC, Bracken M. Meta-analysis of the relationship between asymptomatic bacteriuria and preterm delivery/low birth weight. Obstet Gynecol. 1989;73:576–82.
15. Rouse DJ, Andrews WW, Goldenberg RL, Owen J. Screening and treatment of asymptomatic bacteriuria of pregnancy to prevent pyelonephritis: a cost-effectiveness and cost-benefit analysis. Obstet Gynecol. 1995;86:119–23.
16. Bachman JW, Heise RH, Naessens JM, Timmerman MG. A study of various tests to detect asymptomatic urinary tract infections in an obstetric population. JAMA. 1993;270:1971–4.

17. Mathai E, Thomas RJ, Chandy S, Mathai M, Bergstrom S., Antimicrobials for the treatment of urinary tract infection in pregnancy: practices in southern India.,Pharmacoepidemiol Drug Saf. 2004 Sep;13(9):645–52.

18. Peddie BA, Bailey RR, Wells JE. Resistance of urinary tract isolates of *Escherichia coli* to cotrimoxazole, sulphonamide, trimethoprim and ampicillin: An 11-year survey. N Z Med J. 1987;100:341–2.

19. Sanders CC, Sanders WE Jr. Beta-lactam resistance in gram-negative bacteria: Global trends and clinical impact. Clin Infect Dis. 1992;15:824–3.

20. Vazquez JC, Villar J. Treatments for symptomatic urinary tract infections during pregnancy. Cochrane Database Syst Rev. 2003(4):CD002256.

21. Smaill F. Antibiotics for asymptomatic bacteriuria in pregnancy. Cochrane Database Syst Rev. 2001(2):CD000490.

22. Fihn SD. Clinical practice. Acute uncomplicated urinary tract infection in women. N Engl J Med. 2003;349:259–266.

23. Villar J, Lydon-Rochelle MT, Gulmezoglu AM, Roganti A. Duration of treatment for asymptomatic bacteriuria during pregnancy. Cochrane Database Syst Rev. 2000(2):CD000491.

24. Gupta K, Trautner BW, Urinary Tract Infections, Pyelonephritis, and Prostatitis, Harrison's Principles of Internal Medicine. 18th Ed.p 2394.

25. Millar LK, Wing DA, Paul RH, Grimes DA. Outpatient treatment of pyelonephritis in pregnancy: A randomized controlled trial. Obstet Gynecol. Oct 1995;86(4 Pt 1):560–4.

26. Mead PJ, Harris RE. The incidence of group B beta hemolytic streptococcus in antepartum urinary tract infections. Obstet Gynecol. 1978;51:412–4.

27. Pass MA, Gray BM, Dillon HC Jr. Puerperal and perinatal infections with group B streptococci. Am J Obstet Gynecol. 1982;143:147–52.

28. Victoria M. Allen, Mark H. Yudin, Management of Group B Streptococcal Bacteriuria in Pregnancy, J ObstetGynaecol Can 2012;34(5):482–486.

29. Pfau A, Sacks TG. Effective prophylaxis for recurrent urinary tract infections during pregnancy. Clin Infect Dis. 1992;14:810–4.

13

Respiratory Infections in Pregnancy

Sanjay W Gulhane, Dhananjay Ogale

INTRODUCTION

Pregnancy produces profound changes in the body of a female. Similarly respiratory system of a pregnant female undergoes a lot of changes. Respiratory tissues, anatomical relationships, and respiratory function are altered by the gravid uterus and the hormonal and metabolic changes of advancing gestation.[1,2] It is very important to interpret the laboratory data keeping these changes in mind.

"The commonest of these respiratory infections is pneumonia". The incidence of pneumonia has been estimated to be around 1.1 to 2.7 per 1000 deliveries.[13,21] This is almost similar to the other non-pregnant population.

ANATOMICAL CHANGES IN RESPIRATORY TRACT DURING PREGNANCY

Upper Respiratory Tract

The upper respiratory mucosa during pregnancy reveals hyperaemia, glandular hyperactivity, increased phagocytic activity, and increased mucopolysaccharide content.

Lower Respiratory Tract

Changes in thorax and abdomen are observed even before significant distension of uterus. The subcostal angle increases from 68 degrees to up to 103 degrees.[3,4] The diaphragm rises by up to 4 cm, and the chest diameter can increase up to 2 cm or more,[1,5,6] this leads to 'barrel shaped chest'. Increase in blood volume by almost 40% and decrease in oncotic pressure of the blood lead to increase in pulmonary fluid content.

PHYSIOLOGICAL CHANGES DURING PREGNANCY

Physiological changes during pregnancy include increased respiratory secretions, increased blood volume leading to plethora. Because the diaphragm is displaced upward, there is a decrease in 'residual volume' and 'expiratory reserve volume', resulting in a decreased 'functional residual capacity'. Conversely, inspiratory capacity and tidal volume increase, so that 'vital capacity' and 'total lung capacity' remain the same.[5,6]

IMMUNOLOGICAL CHANGES DURING PREGNANCY

Alterations in cellular immunity have been widely reported and are aimed primarily at protecting the foetus from the mother. These changes include decreased lymphocyte proliferative response, especially in the second and third trimesters, decreased natural killer cell activity, changes in T cell populations with a decrease in numbers of circulating helper T cells, reduced lymphocyte cytotoxic activity, and production by the trophoblast of substances that could block maternal recognition of fetal major histocompatibility antigens.[7,8]

In addition, hormones prevalent during pregnancy—including progesterone, human chorionic gonadotropin, alpha-fetoprotein and cortisol—may inhibit cell mediated immune function.These changes could theoretically increase the risk from infection, particularly by viral and fungal pathogens.[9,10]

SYMPTOMATOLOGY OF RESPIRATORY INFECTIONS

The common symptoms can be listed as follows:

- Cough is the commonest symptom.
- Dyspnoea
- Fever
- Nasal discharge
- The other symptoms are haemoptysis, chest pain.
- These are not different than general populations.

UPPER RESPIRATORY INFECTIONS

The upper respiratory infections occur with similar frequency in pregnancy as in common population.

- *Rhinitis:* Inflammation of the nasal mucosa
- *Rhinosinusitis or sinusitis:* Inflammation of the nares and paranasal sinuses, including frontal, ethmoid, maxillary, and sphenoid
- *Nasopharyngitis (rhinopharyngitis or the common cold):* Inflammation of the nares, pharynx, hypopharynx, uvula, and tonsils
- *Pharyngitis:* Inflammation of the pharynx, hypopharynx, uvula, and tonsils
- *Epiglottitis (supraglottitis):* Inflammation of the superior portion of the larynx and supraglottic area
- *Laryngitis:* Inflammation of the larynx
- *Laryngotracheitis:* Inflammation of the larynx, trachea, and subglottic area
- *Tracheitis:* Inflammation of the trachea and subglottic area.

- *Aetiology:* The commonest organisms causing Upper respiratory infections are viruses. The most common viruses are:
  - Rhinoviruses
  - Coronaviruses
  - Adenoviruses
  - Coxsackieviruses
  - Influenza viruses.

Bacterial causes of pharyngitis include the following:
- Group A streptococci
- Group C and G streptococci
- *Neisseria gonorrhoeae*
- *Arcanobacterium (Corynebacterium) hemolyticum*
- *Corynebacterium diphtheriae*
- Atypical bacteria (e.g. Mycoplasma pneumoniae and Chlamydia pneumoniae; absent lower respiratory tract disease, the clinical significance of these pathogens is uncertain)
- Anaerobicbacteria.

Complications of upper respiratory tract infections:
- Otitis media
- Bronchitis
- Bronchiolitis
- Pneumonia
- Sepsis
- Meningitis
- Intracranial abscess
- Rheumatic fever with heart disease.

Diagnosis of Upper Respiratory Tract Infections

Testing of nasopharyngeal specimen is needed when looking for a specific organism. Diagnosis of specific disorders is based on the following tests:

- *Group A streptococcal infection:* Clinical findings or a history of exposure to a case, supported by results of rapid-detection assays and cultures (positive rapid antigen detection tests do not necessitate a backup culture)

- *Acute bacterial rhinosinusitis:* Laboratory studies are generally not indicated; Computed tomography (CT) scanning or other sinus imaging may be appropriate if symptoms persist despite therapy or if complications (e.g. extension of disease into surrounding tissue) are suspected.
- *Influenza:* Rapid tests have over 70% sensitivity and more than 90% specificity.
- *Mononucleosis:* Heterophile antibody testing (e.g. Monospot).
- *Herpes simplex virus infection:* Cell culture or polymerase chain reaction (PCR) assay.
- *Pertussis:* Rapid tests; culture of a nasopharyngeal aspirate (criterion standard).
- *Epiglottitis:* Direct visualization by laryngoscopy, performed by an otorhinolaryngologist.
- *Gonococcal pharyngitis:* Gram staining of nasal secretions and throat culture for *Neisseria gonorrhoeae.*
- *H1N1 influenza:* Throat swab with PCR of the sample.

Treatment of Upper Respiratory Infections

The mild viral infections need only supportive therapy in the form of decongestants, anti-inflammatory drugs and antipyretics.

The community acquired mild bacterial infections respond to antibiotics like amoxycillin, amoxycillin and clavulanic acid combination, azithromycine, cephalosporins.

Group A Streptococcal Disease

- Oral penicillin or amoxicillin for 10 days for patients without an allergy to penicillin.
- If compliance is a concern, consider a single intra-muscular injection of benzathine penicillin G.
- A first-generation cephalosporin may be used in patients with non-anaphylactic penicillin allergy.
- Options for penicillin-allergic patients include Clindamycin or Clarithromycin for 10 days or Azithromycin for 5 days.[11]

LOWER RESPIRATORY TRACT INFECTIONS

Community acquired pneumonia (CAP) is recognised as a most common non-obstetric infection that carries a substantial risk of maternal and foetal morbidity and mortality in peripartum period.

No significant differences in maternal age and parity have been identified between women who have pneumonia during pregnancy and those who do not.[12] Mean gestational age at admission for pneumonia ranges from 24 to 31 weeks.[12,13] First trimester is the period with lowest risk of pneumonia during pregnancy.

Symptoms: Cough (productive or non-productive), fever, dyspnoea, pleuritic chest pain, haemoptysis are commonly seen and helps to establish the diagnosis. But misdiagnosis is very common and has been observed in studies done by Yost *et al*[12] and Madinger *et al.*[13]

Risk Factors

1. *Anemia:* Benedetti *et al*[14] in their study noted that Hb <10 gm was a risk factor for developing pneumonia. But this finding was not supported by another study done by Richey *et al.*[15]
2. Asthma.[16]
3. Antepartum use of steroids to improve fetal lung maturity.[17]
4. Tocolytic agents given to induce labour have been associated with the development of pneumonia. It has been said that these agents lead to pulmonary edema and increase the risk.[18,19]
5. Smoking.[20]

Pathogens: The organisms causing pneumonia are same as that in non-pregnant population. The relative percentages of various pathogens are mentioned in Table 13.1.

Legionella pneumonia is very uncommon but can be a cause of very serious disease. Legionella can present as typical or atypical pneumonia.

Table 13.1: Pathogens implicated in pneumonia during pregnancy: From four studies (n=161)[13,14,15,21]

Pathogen	no (%)
Streptococcus pneumoniae	28 (17%)
Haemophilus influenzae	9 (5.5%)
Mycoplasma pneumoniae	5 (3%)
Legionella sp.	2 (1.2%)
Staphylococcus aureus	2 (1.2%)
Influenza A virus	2 (1.2%)
Others	14 (9%)
Unknown	99 (61%)

Aspiration of the gastric contents can lead to aspiration pneumonia as pregnant females are prone for aspiration due to decreased oesophageal tone, elevation of diaphragm and enlarging gravid uterus. In such condition anaerobic organisms can cause pulmonary infections.

Viruses: Influenza viruses A, B, C, and Varicella are most common. Other viruses are rubeola, infectious mononucleosis, Hanta virus.

Highest mortality with influenza has been found in 3rd trimester of pregnancy.[22]

Fungi: Fungal infection, notably coccidioidomycosis, may rarely complicate pregnancy. This may be because of the defects in cell-mediated immunity during the pregnancy. Cryptococcal infection and blastomycosis are rare infections.

HIV and respiratory infections in pregnancy: Pneumocystis jirovici occurs at very high rate in pregnant females with HIV infection. Co-trimoxozole is the drug of choice. Pentamidine, clindamycin and primaquin are the alternatives.

Diagnosis and Investigations

- A thorough history and detailed examination of respiratory system of the patient is often enough to clinically diagnose pneumonia.
- *Blood investigations*
  - Complete blood count.
  - Blood culture.
  - Sputum examination with gram and AFB staining and culture.

Other investigations like liver and renal functions should also be obtained.

- *Chest X-ray:* It is safe during pregnancy as it does not exceed the maximum advisable limit of radiation to the fetus, i.e. 5 rad. As per the guidelines for diagnostic imaging during pregnancy given by American Congress of Obstetricians and Gynecologists, 2 views of chest X ray lead to 0.02–0.07 mrad which is very low and not an indication for abortion or chest X-ray can be obtained with abdominal lead shield (Figs 13.1 and 13.2).

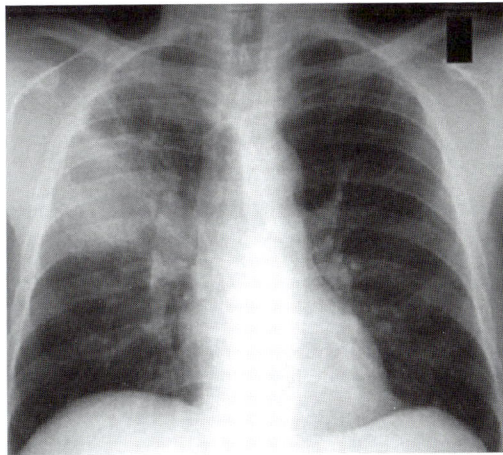

Fig. 13.1: Lobar pneumonia

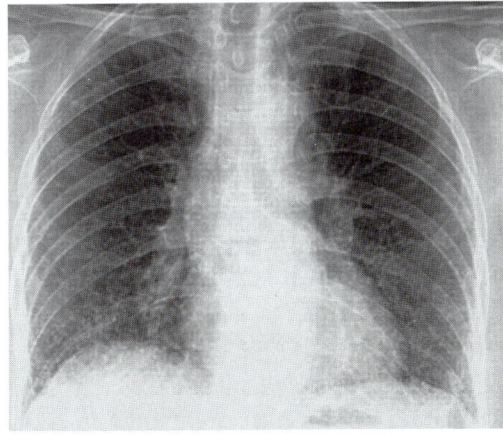

Fig. 13.2: Interstitial pneumonia

TREATMENT OF COMMUNITY ACQUIRED PNEUMONIA IN PREGNANCY

- Propped up position.
- Supportive treatment with intravenous fluids.
- Nasal oxygen inhalation according to blood gas or pulse oxymetry reports.
- Nebulisation with bronchodilators as and when indicated.
- Non-invasive and invasive ventilatory support in severely hypoxic patients.
- Inotropic support.

The commonly used agents are:

- Cephalosporins—cefriaxone 1gm bid/ Cefotaxime 1 gm tid for intravenous use
- Cefixime 200 mg bid/cefuroxime 500 mg bid/Cefadroxil for oral use.
- Penicillins—amoxycillin + clavulanic acid 1.2 gm bid for intravenous or 625 mg for oral use.
- Crystalline penicillin can also be used.
- Macrolides—azithromycine 500 mg once a day for either intravenous or oral use, erythromycine, clindamycine and clarithromycine can be used as alternatives.
- Penems (meropenem, imipenem + cilastatin, doripenem) should be used in seriously ill patients with gram negative pneumonias (especially Pseudomonas).
- Antivirals—acyclovir 800 mg 5 times/day orally or 500 mg tid intravenously can be used for suspected cases of viral pneumonia.
- Antifungals—should be used judiciously in fungal pneumonias. Co-trimoxozole is reserved for pneumocystis pneumonia in immunocompromised hosts.

Criteria for indoor therapy: CURB 65 criteria are very useful for this purpose.[23,24]

TUBERCULOSIS IN PREGNANCY

Pulmonary tuberculosis is a very commonly found lung infection in pregnancy in India. Such patients are investigated with chest radiographs and sputum examination similar to non-pregnant population. The four standard drugs used are Rifampicin, Isoniazid, Ethambutol and Pyrizinamide. Streptomycin is added in relapse of disease or failure of treatment or in defaulters. Streptomycin is pregnancy category D drug and known to cause damage to eighth cranial nerve. So should be used when benefits outweigh the risks to the mother.

The patients are treated with the standard anti-tubercular drugs as per the National guidelines (DOTS) irrespective of the period of gestation.

H1N1 (SWINE FLU)

This needs a special mention as pregnant females are thought to be more susceptible to infection with H1N1 virus. Pregnant patients with H1N1 infection are considered Category B-2 patients.

Diagnosis is made by Reverse Transcriptase-Polymerase Chain Reaction (RT-PCR) test of the sample of throat secretions obtained by throat swab of suspected patients.

Treatment

As per the guidelines issued by Ministry of Health and Family Welfare of India 'Oseltamavir' is the drug of choice for H1N1 infection. Dose of the drug is 75 mg bid for 5 days. The dose for prophylaxis is 75 mg OD for 10 days. This drug should be used during pregnancy only if the benefit outweighs the risk to the foetus.

CONCLUSION

Pregnancy leads to significant anatomical and physiological changes in body and is also an immunosuppressed state. This makes all pregnant females susceptible to various infections and also increase the morbidity and mortality in pregnancy. Respiratory infections are one of the common amongst them and occur with same incidence as the non-pregnant population. Upper and lower

Table 13.2: Safety in pregnancy of selected antimicrobial agents commonly used to treat pneumonias

Class of antibiotic	Evidence regarding adverse effects	Safety in pregnancy
Penicillins	Widely used without evidence of problems	Good
Cephalosporins	Widely used without evidence of problems	Good
Macrolides	Widely used without evidence of problems. Most information relates to erythromycin and less to clarithromycin or azithromycin	Good
Aminoglycosides	No published reports on fetal nephropathy after maternal gentamicin, however, ability of premature infants to eliminate gentamicin seems to be dependent on gestational age.	Potential risk of nephropathy and ototoxicity. Maternal plasma levels should be carefully monitored if clear indication exists for its use
Sulphonamides	May cause kernicterus if given in late pregnancy. Of 2296 newborns exposed to co-trimoxazole during the first trimester, 126 (5.5%) major birth defects were observed, 98 expected.	Avoid. Insufficient information on high doses. Theoretical risk of neural tube defects with co-trimoxazole due to its folate antagonist activity
Quinolones	Arthralgia and tendonitis reported in adults but none following in utero exposure in human pregnancy.	Insufficient evidence of safety
Tetracyclines	Administration in the second or third trimesters can cause yellow-brown staining and banding of the teeth of the child and reversible growth retardation of the long bones.	Avoid, especially at or after 12 weeks
Metronidazole	Conflicting data. Some epidemiological studies suggest increased risk of malformations, still-births and low birth weight infants. Other studies totalling exposure to over 3000 newborns have found no increase in congenital anomalies.	Unclear
Antiviral agents		
Amantadine	Limited preclinical data in animals showed a possible association with cleft palate. In a study of 64 pregnancies, five births with defects were reported.	Insufficient evidence of safety
Ribavirin	Teratogenic or embryolethal in nearly all animal species	Avoid
Acyclovir	Prospective register (1984–99) with data on 1246 pregnancies showed no increase in birth defects compared with the general population (GlaxoWellcome Medical Information, personal communication)	Use recommended in situations where risk from untreated infection is greater than risk of possible adverse effects, e.g. life threatening varicella infections
Antifungal agents		
Amphotericin B	Case reports of fetal toxicity involving anemia, transient acidosis with uraemia, and respiratory failure.	Use if benefit outweighs risk of fetal toxicity (usually maternal toxicity also present)
Itraconazole	Embryo-toxic and teratogenic in laboratory animals. 95 of 198 women exposed during the first trimester, 3.2% major malformations were seen.	Best avoided. Manufacturer recommends contraception during and for one menstrual cycle after stopping treatment
Fluconazole	Embryo-toxic and teratogenic in high doses in rats. Multiple congenital abnormalities reported with high dose use in humans. Possible dose dependent teratogenicity.	Avoid

respiratory infections in pregnancy are diagnosed and treated in similar manner to the non-pregnant population. Single chest X-ray gives very minute dose of radiation to fetus and hence is safe during pregnancy. Antibiotics should be used judiciously in pregnancy, keeping in mind their side effects and risks to the fetus. Tuberculosis is treated with standard four drug therapy in pregnancy. Pregnant patients are found to be high risk for H1N1 infections and should be promptly treated with standard doses of Oseltamavir.

REFERENCES

1. Weinberger SE, Weiss ST, Cohen WR, et al.(1980) State of the art pregnancy and the lung. Am Rev Respir Dis 121:559–581.

2. Azioglu K, Kaltreider NL, Rosen M, et al. (1970) Pulmonary function during pregnancy in normal women and in patients with cardiopulmonary disease. Thorax 25:445–450.

3. The human respiratory nasal mucosa in pregnancy. An electron microscopic and histochemical studyToppozada H, Michaels L, Toppozada M, El-Ghazzawi I, Talaat M, Elwany S J Laryngol Otol. 1982;96(7):613.

4. The chest radiograph in pregnancy. Turner AF, ClinObstet Gynecol. 1975;18(3):65.

5. Cugell DW, Frank NR, Gaensler EA, Badger TL: Pulmonary function in pregnancy: I. Serial observations in normal women. Am Rev Tuberc 67: 568, 1953.

6. Alaily AB, Carrol KB: Pulmonary ventilation in pregnancy. Br J ObstetGynaecol 85: 518, 1978.

7. Baley JE, Schacter BZ (1985) Mechanisms of diminished natural killer cell activity in pregnant women and neonates. J Immunol 134:3042–3048.

8. Bulmer R, Hancock KW (1977) Depletion of circulating T lymphocytes in pregnancy. ClinExpImmunol 28:302–305.

9. Lederman MM (1984) Cell-mediated immunity and pregnancy. Chest 86:6–9S.

10. Sridama V, Pacini F,Yang SL, et al.(1982) Decreased levels of helper T cells: A possible cause of immunodeficiency in pregnancy. N Engl J Med 307:352–356.

11. [Guideline] Shulman ST, Bisno AL, Clegg HW, Gerber MA, Kaplan EL, Lee G, et al. Clinical practice guideline for the diagnosis and management of group A streptococcal pharyngitis: 2012 update by the Infectious Diseases Society of America. Clin Infect Dis. Nov 15 2012;55(10):1279–82.

12. Yost NP,Bloom SL, Richey SD, et al. (2000) An appraisal of treatment guidelines for antepartum community-acquired pneumonia. Am J ObstetGynecol 183:131–135.

13. Madinger NE, Greenspoon JS, Ellrodt AG (1989) Pneumonia during pregnancy: Has modern technology improved maternal and fetal outcome? Am J Obstet Gynecol161:657–662.

14. Benedetti TJ, Valle R, Ledger WJ (1982) Antepartum pneumonia in pregnancy. Am J ObstetGynecol 144:413–417.

15. Richey SD, Roberts SW, Ramin KD, et al. (1994) Pneumonia complicating pregnancy. Obstet Gynecol 84:525–528.

16. Munn MB, Groome LJ, Atterbury JL, et al.(1999) Pneumonia as a complication of pregnancy. J MaternFetal Med 8:151–154.

17. Rotmensch S, Vishne TH, Celentano C, et al.(1999) Maternal infectious morbidity following multiple courses of betamethasone. J Infect 39:49–54.

18. Maccato M(1991) Respiratory insufficiency due to pneumonia in pregnancy. ObstetGynecolClin North Am 18:289–299.

19. Goodrum LA(1997) Pneumonia in pregnancy. SeminPerinatol 21:276–283.

20. Nuorti JP, Butler JC, Farley MM, et al.(2000) Cigarette smoking and invasive pneumococcal disease. Active Bacterial Core Surveillance Team. N Engl J Med342:681–689.

21. Berkowitz K, LaSala A (1990) Risk factors associated with the increasing prevalence of pneumonia during pregnancy. Am J Obstet Gynecol 163:981–985.

22. McKinney WP, Volkert P, Kaufman J(1990) Fatal swine influenza pneumonia during late pregnancy. Arch Intern Med 150:213–215.

23. Lim WS, van der Eerden MM, Laing R, et. al. Defining community acquired pneumonia severity on presentation to hospital: an international derivation and validation study. Thorax. 2003 May;58(5):377–82.

24. Lim WS, Macfarlane JT, Boswell TC, et. al. Study of community acquired pneumonia aetiology (SCAPA) in adults admitted to hospital: implications for management guidelines. Thorax. 2001 Apr;56(4):296–301.

14

Breast Diseases and Fever

Rachna Bhagat, Kartikeya Bhagat

Fever is a distressing complaint, not only for the mother but also for the obstetrician. It can mar the joy of motherhood, especially in the early puerperium. Fever, which would have been ignored in the non-pregnant state, is a cause of panic in the puerperium, more so because of fear of passing the infection to the newborn.

Fever is a symptom and the causes of the underlying disease could be innumerable. Fever could be a sign of inflammation or infection anywhere in the body—be it a local condition like surgical wound, endometritis, breast conditions, systemic diseases like respiratory or urinary tract infection, an incidental parasitic infestation like Malaria or a simple viral fever. Although, the commonest cause of fever in puerperium could be an infective pathology like UTI or URTI, it is not unusual to find an infected surgical wound (episiotomy or a caesarean section wound) or a breast condition. However, malaria other parasitic fevers or a viral fever should always be kept in mind and ruled out.

Once the baby delivers, breastfeeding is of paramount significance. Initiation of breastfeeding should happen within an hour of birth—Breast Crawl is the most natural method of initiation of breastfeeding. Faulty technique of breastfeeding, especially improper 'position' and 'attachment' for breastfeeding will result in a sore or a cracked nipple which will manifest on the second or third day after birth. Cracked nipple is a harbinger of Mastitis or a breast abscess if corrective measures are not taken in time.

The common breast conditions that cause fever are:

1. Engorgement
2. Mastitis and
3. Breast abscess.

We also need to discuss *sore nipple* and the *cracked nipple* as it forms the portal for entry of infection into the breast.

SORE NIPPLES

Breast sensitivity increases after birth and most mothers' complaint about some pain or soreness while breastfeeding. During the early postpartum period many women report pain only when the baby first latches on, lasting for about 20–30 seconds. This is nipple stretching discomfort resulting from a kind of low load muscle strain as nipple tissues adjust to stretching. If the pain subsides once the baby is latched, mother can safely ignore it. Suction and *compression* damage are two primary physical causes of nipple pain. If the soreness persists, the technique of breast-feeding could be at fault and it may progress to a cracked nipple.

CRACKED NIPPLE (Figs 14.1A and B)

- Sore nipple, if neglected, leads to cracked nipple in most cases.

Table 14.1: Mohrbacher system of staging nipple trauma

Stage	Pain	Description
Stage I	Superficial pain	Intact skin (redness, bruising, swelling)
Stage II	Superficial pain	Tissue breakdown (abrasion, shallow fissure, compression stripe, blistering)
Stage III	Pain	Partial thickness erosion (skin breakdown to the lower layers of dermis, deep fissure)
Stage IV	Pain	Full thickness erosion (full erosion through dermis)

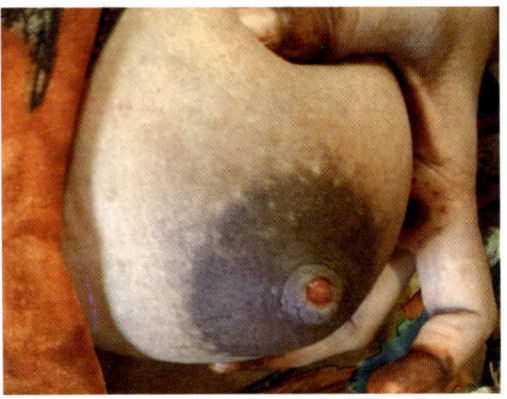

Fig. 14.1A: Cracked nipple-long standing

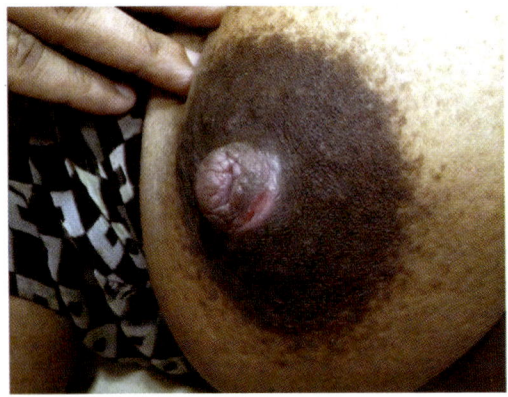

Fig. 14.1B: Circumferential crack

- Cracked nipple is the result of improper technique of breastfeeding: Improper 'latching' or 'attachment' often leads to nipple trauma and cracked nipple.
- If the baby's attachment on the breast is improper, it will bite the nipple with extra force which will further block the milk ducts and cause injury. If the baby is taken off the breast without breaking the suction grip, it can lead to a circumferential crack at the base of the nipple.

- Frequent washing of nipple and areola with soap and water can cause drying and will make the nipples prone to develop cracks by removing the protective natural oily substance which normally covers this area. Routine once a day cleaning of the breasts during bath is sufficient.
- The crack can get secondarily infected and cause mastitis or an abscess.
- The basic treatment is correcting the position/attachment, change the grip, relieve engorgement, instruct the mothers to keep the nipple clean and dry.
- *Treatment of fresh crack:* Nipple wound may be cleaned with warm soapy water once a day, flush the nipple wound with normal saline after each breastfeed to prevent re-colonisation of open crack by pathogens from baby's mouth, air or gently pat dry nipples before applying expressed milk, purified lanolin, local antibiotic cream or hydrogel dressing.
- Nipple shields may be used.
- For severe cases it may be wise to express the milk out to feed the baby with vati-spoon till the crack heals.

FULL BREAST, ENGORGEMENT, MASTITIS AND ABSCESS

- Usually milk 'flows in' by the 3rd or 4th day (usually by 72 hrs) when the mother feels her breasts heavy or full.
- As the milk supply increases, while the demand is still low, the breasts become heavy and engorged.
- If infection sets into the engorged breast, it leads to mastitis.
- When the mastitis is improperly treated, it gets localised to form an abscess.

- Regular breast emptying is the first line of defence against inflammatory breast disorders and failure to remove milk has consequences in terms of not only breast health but also maintenance of adequate milk output.

Full Breast

- Completely filled with milk, just before feeding
- Usually occurs after 3–5 days, is usually bilateral
- Breast is soft, easy to breastfeed, easy to express milk.

Engorgement

Breast is overfilled with milk. Milk, exceeding the storage capacity of the breast tissue, leaks into the interstitial spaces evoking an inflammatory reaction causing pain, mild fever and increasing chances of infection.

Breast becomes hard, skin over the breast is stretched and appears shiny, nipples become flat, shorter and stretched; it could be unilateral or bilateral. Breastfeeding becomes difficult.

Treatment

1. *Symptomic relief:* Anti-inflammatory drugs usually help. Other methods are use of cabbage leaves, ultrasound or acupuncture treatment; however, oxytocin and hot packs are not found to be useful.
2. Gentle massage along the lymphatic drainage pathway improves lymph flow, relieves swelling and improves milk flow. Every mother should be taught the technique of Milk Expression before discharge.
3. *Pharmacological management:* Drugs to suppress milk oversupply may be used judiciously along with massage, etc. Drugs used: Bromergocriptin 1.25 mg as a single dose, to be repeated as required, pseudo-ephidrine 60 mg daily—not to be used in hypertensives.

If engorgement is not relieved, it may progress to mastitis/abscess formation and ultimately result in decreased milk production because of down-regulation.

Mastitis (Fig. 14.2A and B)

Inflammation of breast tissue, usually due to infection (usually through cracks in the nipple), that produces localized tenderness, redness and heat together with systemic reactions of fever, malaise and sometimes nausea and vomiting are hallmarks of mastitis. Varieties range from non-infectious inflammation and sub-clinical mastitis to infectious mastitis and abscess.

Common in the first four weeks post-partum mastitis is typically unilateral with a red, hot, tender swollen wedge-shaped area of the breast, but bilateral mastitis can occur.

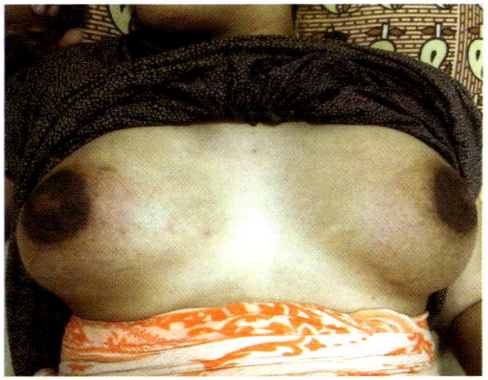

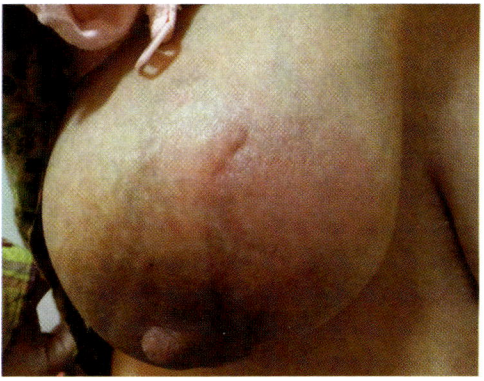

Fig. 14.2A and B: Mastitis

Portal of entry of the disease is through the lactiferous ducts to a secreting lobule, usually thru a cracked nipple to periductal lymphatics or through hematogenous spread. Common organisms involved are *Staphylococcus aureus*, *E. Coli* or other Gram Negative organisms, rarely group A Streptococci, *Streptococcus pneumoniae* and Bacteroides. Streptoccocus infection should be ruled out when mastitis is bilateral.

Predisposing factors: Poor drainage of a duct and an alveolus (engorged breast with insufficient emptying, missing a feed, obstructed duct because of tight clothing), cracked nipple with infection, poor hygiene, lowered immunity associated with stress, fatigue and malnutrition. Treatment includes:

1. Emptying the breast (frequent feeding, regular expression of milk), adequate rest, plenty of fluids.

2. Anti-inflammatory drugs and

3. *Antibiotics:* Commonly used antibiotics include first-generation cephalosporins, ampi-amoxycilian, amox-clavulonic acid or Erythromycin/clindamycin for patients allergic to penicillins/cephalosporins. Suspected MRSA may be treated with vancomycin, clindamycin or rifampicin. Antibiotics should be given for at least 10–14 days as shorter courses are associated with high incidence of relapse.

4. Continue breastfeeding. Infants usually remain well. Sometimes babies refuse breastfeed from a mastitic breast—due to salty taste of milk because of high levels of sodium and chloride. In such cases, ask the mother to discard milk form the affected side and continue feeding from the unaffected side

MRSA should be ruled out when mastitis fails to resolve with front line drug therapy.

Secondary candida infection may occur following prolonged antibiotic use.

Prevention: Proper breastfeeding techniques, early detection and appropriate treatment of mastitis is critical to prevent early weaning, protect infant growth and reduce the risk of transmission of infectious diseases to infants.

Royal college of midwives (2002) recommendations regarding mastitis state: "it might be appropriate to delay antibiotic therapy for 12–24 hours, whilst taking corrective measures to reduce inflammation and promote thorough breast drainage. If however, there was no improvement to this time, a broad spectrum antibiotic would be necessary."

ABM (2008) mastitis protocol (citing the WHO publication) states that if there is no positive response to antibiotics within two days, if the mastitis reoccurs, if it is hospital-acquired mastitis or if it is severe or unusual, breast milk culture or sensitivity testing should be done.

Mothers pumping for a sick or premature baby should be directed to discard the milk from the mastitc breast until symptoms resolve. (Neifert 1999, Behari 2004).

BREAST ABSCESS (Figs 14.3, 14.4A to C)

Breast abscesses are pus filled cysts that develop as a consequence of unresolved/untreated/inadequately treated mastitis.

Abscesses are more common in primiparous women, older women and those who give birth postmaturely. The risk is increased if abrupt weaning occurs following mastitis, antibiotic therapy is delayed, wrong antibiotic

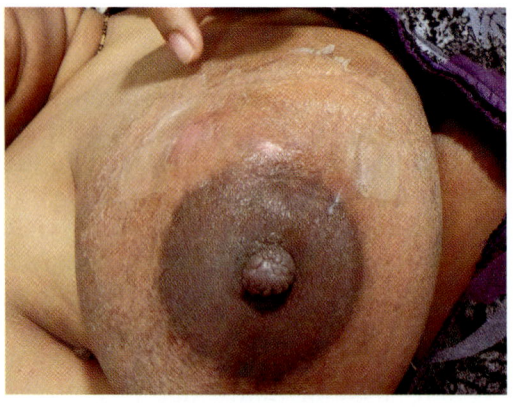

Flig 14.3: Breast abscess

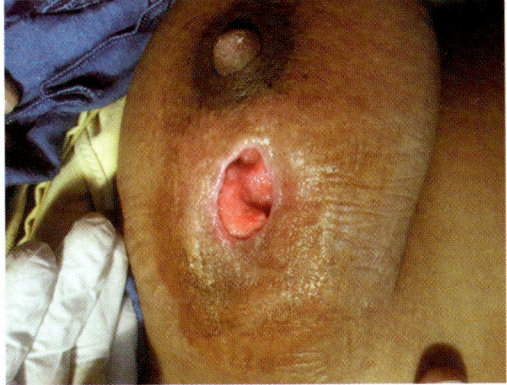

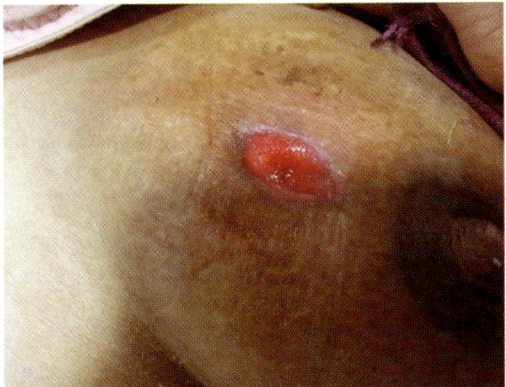

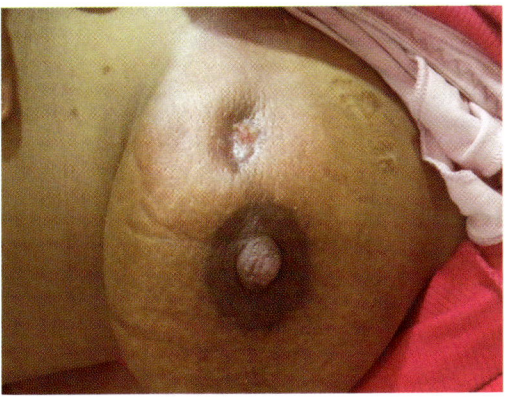

Fig. 14.4A to C: Breast Abscess: healing process after I&D

breast abscesses come in myriad of sizes, different positions in the breast, may be superficial or deep, overlying skin is usually inflamed-red and at times the abscess may be pointing. Ultrasonography may be used to confirm the diagnosis and define the size.

Apart from antimicrobials and anti-inflammatory drugs, the standard treatment is incision and drainage (I&D) of the abscess. However, recovery from I&D in a lactating breast is usually slow, may take 4–6 weeks. The incision needs to be kept open and draining till the wound fills up with granulation tissue from within. If the wound heals too quickly, fistulas may form; the open wound will leak milk continuously, pain could be unbearable; dressing the wound would be messy, cumbersome and the whole appearance ghastly to the woman and the family. Keeping the skin dry may help to prevent maceration in the surrounding area and skin breakdown. The procedure may be done under local or general anaesthesia, increasing the risk. The mother, invariably, ends up with stopping breastfeeding.

Aspiration of the breast abscess (Fig. 14.5A, B, C) is a very good baby-friendly alternative to the standard I&D procedure—it is simple, easy to perform, much less invasive, performed under local anaesthesia, does not require regular dressings, avoids all the grotesque consequences of the I&D and is equally effective. More than anything else, needle aspiration allows uninterrupted continued breastfeeding. The procedure may be performed under USG guidance.

Procedure

- Counseling the patient and the family about the procedure, advantages over I&D, continuing breastfeeding, need for multiple sittings for a large abscess.
- Confirm the diagnosis: Size, site
- Consent
- Part painted and draped

is used or if the woman fails to complete the full course of antibiotic.

Typically, the history would be engorgement not responding to conservative treatment, increased pain and redness in the breast followed by fever and a well defined lump in the breast. Cracked nipple may be present.

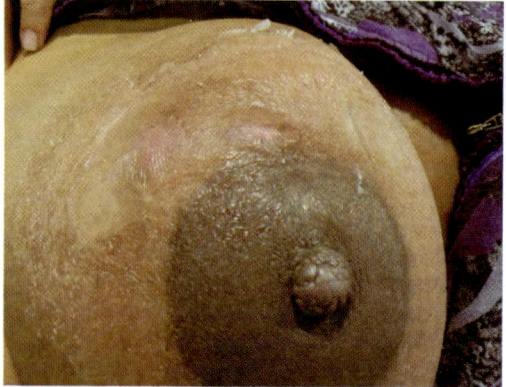

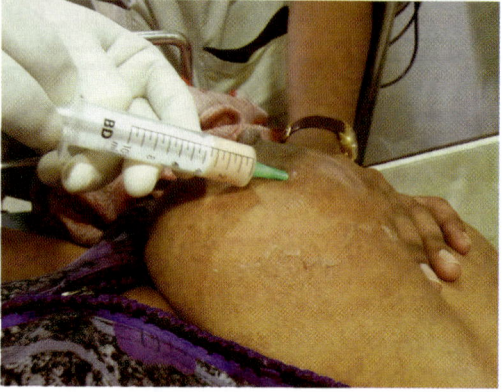

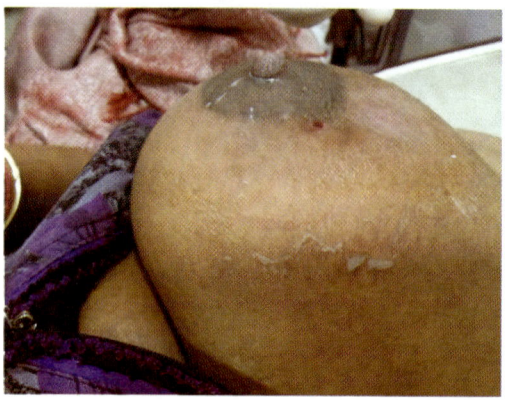

Fig. 14.5: Breast abscess: Technique of aspiration

- *Site of aspiration:* The most superficial part of the abscess or the site where the abscess is pointing.
- Inject 1% local anesthetic at the site of aspiration and inside the abscess cavity.
- Puncture the abscess with a 16 gauge needle and aspirate the contents—the contents may be sent for culture. Break all the septa inside the cavity with the needle. Aspirate as much pus as possible. You may irrigate the cavity with normal saline or dilute betadine solution to remove all the purulent material from the cyst. The procedure may have to be repeated a couple of times if the abscess reforms, especially if it is big. For large abscesses (> 3 cm), catheter drains may be placed for continuous drainage, decreasing the need for multiple aspirations and surgical incision. The procedure may be performed under USG control.
- The patient can breastfeed the child immediately after the aspiration and go home. The milk remains clean unless the abscess ruptures into the duct system.
- Reconfirm proper 'latching', the mother should know the proper technique of attachment, position and expression of milk.
- Do not clean the baby's mouth as it leads to injuries and persistent infection which may be transferred to the mother during breastfeeding.

APPROACH TO A PATIENT WITH FEVER IN EARLY PUERPERIUM

Principle: To diagnose the breast condition, rule out other causes of fever and then treat the specific Breast condition - keeping in mind the paramount need to continue breastfeeding.

1. History

- *Fever:* Onset, duration, frequency, degree: mild or high fever, with or without chills, associated systemic complaints: burning or frequency of urination; cough with or without expectoration, breathlessness or wheezing and history of use of medications like misoprostol.

Fever associated with breast engorgement would be mild or low grade, persistent and usually without chills. There will not be any other systemic complaints and local

Table 14.2: Signs of inflammatory breast conditions

	Full breast	Engorgement	Mastitis	Abscess
Uni or bilateral	Bilateral	Usually bilateral	Unilateral	Unilateral
Redness	–	+	++	
Particular part	++/+			
Fever	–	+/– (if persist for24 hours)	++	++/+/–
Pain	–	+	++	++/+
Ease of expression	Easy	Difficult	Difficult	Easy From other parts

Table 14.3: Interventions

	Full breast	Engorgement	Mastitis	Abscess
Rest	+	++	+++	+++/++
Analgesics	–	+	++	++/+/–
Antibiotics	–	–	+	+
Emptying of breast	+	+	+	+
Use of cabbage leaves	–	+	–	–
Incision and drainage	–	–	–	+

examination will clinch the diagnosis. However, a thorough examination is warranted to rule out other causes of fever. Typically, tablet misoprostol, especially if used per rectally in the postpartum period, may give rise to fever. If the breast develops mastitis, the fever will persist—may be with chills—and localising signs develop: A sector in the breast will appear red, warm, firm, inflamed and tender may be with a blocked duct opening or a cracked nipple. Left untreated or if treated incompletely.

- *Breastfeeding history:* When did she feel fullness in the breasts, how long did she have engorgement, how often does the baby breastfeed, since when is she finding it difficult to breastfeed, since when does she have pain?

  Typically, a mother feels fullness in the breasts on day 2 or 3 after delivery which progresses to engorgement in a day or two. The nipples become short, firm and the baby finds it difficult to breastfeed. The cracks in the nipple appear by now making breastfeeding all the more difficult and painful. Left untreated, sector mastitis develops which may progress to an abscess or an antibioma.

- History suggesting involvement of other systems like:
  - Frequency and dysuria suggesting UTI
  - Cough with or without expectoration, breathlessness suggesting URTI
  - Periodic fever with chills with signs suggesting malarial infection

2. Examination

- *Confirm the diagnosis:* Check temperature with a thermometer. Fever is considered to be significant only if it is high and persistent
- *Check the general condition of the patient:* Toxic look and pallor may signify serious infection.
- *Local examination:*
  - Breast examination: cracked nipple, firm tender breast with signs of inflammation or an abscess
  - Check the surgical wound (episiotomy or LSCS wound) for signs of infection
  - Check the uterus for signs of sub-involution and endometritis
- *Systemic examination:*
  - Fever, tachycardia, toxic look
  - RS/CVS/renal angle tenderness/palpable liver

3. Investigations

- No investigations required to treat engorged breasts
- To be ordered if fever persists after treating the preliminary breast conditions and the diagnosis/ cause of fever doubtful
- CBC, ESR, PS for MP, urine routine, BUN, SGPT

4. Treatment

- Check the technique of breastfeeding: proper 'attachment', 'position' and 'expression' of milk
- Expression of milk—manual, use of pumps
- Treatment of cracked nipples
- *Drugs:* Anti-inflammatory, antimicrobials
- Surgical treatment of the breast abscess

OUR EXPERIENCE

Fever is not a very common complication one encounters during puerperium. However, any fever in the puerperium should be investigated thoroughly because of possible serious complications in the mother and the baby. Engorgement is the most common breast condition encountered in puerperium. Technique of breast milk expression should be taught to all the mothers before discharge from the hospital and the use of cold compresses or the cabbage leaves should be encouraged. Fever comes up if engorgement is not resolved fast. Cracked nipples occur because of faulty breastfeeding technique. Engorgement coupled with cracked nipples leads to development of mastitis, which if left untreated, develops into a breast abscess. The most appropriate technique of treating the breast abscess is needle aspiration with or without USG guidance. The underlying principle in treating all the breast conditions is to encourage and continue breastfeeding. To tackle the breast and nipple problems effectively post delivery, BFHI and the Ten Steps to successful breastfeeding should be the guiding principles of the maternity service for it to fulfil its role completely.

BIBLIOGRAPHY

1. The Breastfeeding Atlas, 4th edition, Wilson-Clay and Hoover, LactNews Press, USA.
2. Breastfeeding—A Guide for Medical Professionals, 6th edition, Ruth Lawrence and Robert Lawrence, Elsiever Mosby.
3. Ten Steps to Successful Breastfeeding. Protecting, Promoting and Supporting Breastfeeding: The Special Role of Maternity Services, a joint WHO/ UNICEF statement published by the World Health Organization.
4. Evidence for the Ten Steps to Successful Breastfeeding, WHO, 1998.
5. IYCN Modules Level I, II, III created by BPNI (Breastfeeding Promotion Network of India).

15

Cesarean Section and Fever

Arun Nayak, Madhuri Mehendale

INTRODUCTION

A cesarean section has become an extremely safe operation over the years. Most of the serious complications associated with cesarean sections are not usually due to the operation itself. Instead, the complications come from the indication for the cesarean section as well as other associated conditions during the cesarean.

Febrile morbidity is not very uncommon after cesarean delivery. Many variables can alter this risk.

Many complications of cesarean section delivery are unpredictable and very rare, but there are some factors that make women more susceptible to develop complications. These **risk factors**[1] include:

- Prolonged ruptured membranes
- Prolonged labor
- Emergency intrapartum surgery
- Multiple vaginal examinations
- Use of invasive monitoring like fetal scalp electrodes
- Bacterial vaginosis
- Maternal obesity (for wound infections in particular)
- Maternal disease (diabetes, pre-eclampsia, anemia)

PUERPERAL OR POSTPARTUM FEVER AND SEPSIS

Up to 8 percent of women who have a C-section delivery develop a bacterial infection called puerperal fever or postpartum fever (Barrett, 2002). This infection often starts in the uterus or vagina. If it spreads throughout the body, it is called sepsis. Most of the time, the infection is diagnosed early. It can usually be cured with antibiotics. If the infection is untreated and sepsis occurs, it is harder to treat. In rare cases, sepsis can be life threatening. A fever in the first 10 days after the C-section is a warning sign for puerperal sepsis. Infections like urinary tract infections or mastitis (infections in the breasts) can be a sign of this complication. They should be treated quickly to avoid the spread of the infection. Various **types of febrile morbidity** reported are:

- *Endomyometritis:* Depending on the population studied, endometritis may occur in anywhere between 5 and 75 percent of women who have a cesarean section. In the US, 2–15 percent of C-sections result in endometritis (ACOG, 2010)

- *Wound infection:* Reported wound infection rates associated with cesarean section range from 2.5% to 16.1%. Nielson and Hokegard found rates of 4.7% for elective cases and 24.2% for emergency cases.

- Urinary tract infection are a common complication of cesarean section and occur with a variable frequency of 2 to 6%, the rate depending on the duration of catheterisation and the preoperative health of the women.

- Mastitis and breast abscess
- Pelvic parametritis, abscesses are rare

ENDOMYOMETRITIS

- Risk factors for metritis—young maternal age, low socioeconomic status, extended duration of labor, prolonged rupture of membranes, and multiple vaginal examinations.
- In 10% cases, concurrent bacteraemia will accompany postcesarean endomyometritis. Postcesarean endomyometritis is a polymicrobial infection with bacteria normally present in the lower genital tract: aerobic streptococci(group B and D), anaerobic gram positive cocci (peptococcus and peptostreptococcus), aerobic (*E. coli*, *Klebsiella pneumoniae*, Proteus spp.) and anerobic gram negative bacilli (Bacteroides spp. and *Gardenerella vaginalis*).
- Clinical manifestations—fever (excess of 38°C, between 24 and 36 hours of delivery), tachycardia, lower abdominal pain, uterine and adnexal tenderness, and peritoneal irritation, foul lochia and general malaise. Controversy exists as to whether temperature elevations within 24 hrs are pathologic, as can be due to benign causes like overheating due to labour efforts or milk fever.
- Differential diagnosis—mastitis, urinary tract infections, atelectasis and bacterial or viral infections virtually anywhere within the respiratory, genitourinary, and gastrointestinal tracts.
- Examination—breasts, sinuses percussed, lungs and heart auscultated to discover any condition unrelated to uterus. Manual examination and visual inspection of vagina and cervix must be done.
- Laboratory tests—except CBC and urine examination generally not helpful.

Controversy exists about endometrial cultures are helpful prior to starting therapy. If endometrial cultures attempted, some data support use of multiple lumen catheters in order to avoid vaginal contamination.

- *Several effective regimens are available:* Clindamycin (900 mg IV every 8 hrly) plus an aminoglycoside (gentamycin, 1.5 mg/kg IV every 8 hrly)–cure rates of 90% to 97% reported. Most show response in 24 to 48 hrs. treatment, oral antibiotic therapy thereafter generally not necessary, except in staphylococcal bacteraemia. Parenteral therapy stopped after patient is asymptomatic for 24 to 48 hrs. If no response for 48 to 72 hours, modify therapy. Cultures may prove valuable. Resistant organisms like enterococci may be responsible. Adding ampicillin (2 gm IV every 4 hrs) may improve response rate. Failure could be due to concurrent wound infections, drug fever, and pelvic abscess.

WOUND INFECTION

- Risk factors—anemia, premature rupture of membranes, prolapsed cord, and meconium staining.
- Organisms—mixture of aerobic and anaerobic bacteria (*E. coli*, *proteus mirabilis*, Bacteroides spp., beta hemolytic streptococci) are isolated from postcesarean wound infections. 25% of times, *Staphylococcus aureus* is isolated and appears to originate from skin rather than endometrium.
- Management—prompt recognition and treatment is essential. Infected wound is characterised by localised pain, tenderness, erythema, and purulent discharge, typically becoming clinically evident 4 to 7 days after surgery. Fever and leucocytosis may be present.

Initial treatment involves opening the wound along the affected area to the fascia and culturing the exudates. Incision and Drainage with debridement of necrotic tissue is vital. Application of hydrogen peroxide to chemically debride the area should follow initial local surgical efforts. As antiseptic solutions are cytotoxic, saline lavage must follow their application, then wet-to-dry dressing. Once all necrotic tissue is removed and a healthy granulation tissue is formed, wound can be reapproximated or left for secondary intention healing.

- Complication—necrotizing fascitis. Repeated aggressive debridement in association with broad spectrum antibiotics and hyperbaric oxygen therapy is vital to achieve cure.

URINARY TRACT INFECTIONS

- Risk factors—frequent vaginal examinations, urethral catheterization, 5 to 10% incidence of asymptomatic bacteriuria during pregnancy. Other risk factors are unmarried status, cesarean delivery, tocolysis, renal disease, preeclampsia-eclampsia, and abruption placenta.
- Organisms—*Escherichia coli*, *Klebsiella pneumoniae*, and proteus species.
- Complication—pyelonephritis is a serious infection in pregnancy. Can be complicated by ARDS, bacteremia.
- Management—culture urine; appropriate antibiotics (oral or parenteral depending on clinical severity).

INFECTION PROPHYLAXIS

Randomized trials have demonstrated, a single dose of antimicrobial agent given at the time of cesarean delivery will serve to decrease infectious morbidity significantly. This is true for high-risk laboring patients as well as those undergoing elective cesarean delivery (American College of Obstetricians and Gynecologists, 2003).

For women in labor or with ruptured membranes, most recommend a single 2 gm dose of a beta lactum drug—either a cephalosporin or extended spectrum penicillin—after delivery of newborn. This reduces rate of pelvic infection by 70–80% and abdominal incision infections to less than 2%. Prenatal treatment of asymptomatic vaginal infections has not shown to prevent postpartum pelvic infections.

Other measures to reduce infection and hence febrile morbidity[2]

- Meticulous hemostasis—prevents nidus of infection on blood clots
- Good surgical technique
- Preoperative skin preparation
- Clipping hair rather than shaving
- Avoid manual removal of placenta
- Close Camper's fascia
- Limiting number of people in theatre
- Reporting of cases

MORTALITY/MORBIDITY

The prognosis for postpartum infections and fever is good with prompt and appropriate therapy.

In most reviews, maternal death rates associated with infection range from 4 to 8%, or approximately 0.6 maternal deaths per 100,000 live births.

The significant complications associated with cesarean section include the following:

- Scarring
- Infertility
- Sepsis
- Septic shock
- Death

SUMMARY

- Surveillance for normal recovery following cesarean section and dealing with minor complaints is all the majority of women require.
- A few, especially the one with high risk factors, may develop significant problems like postpartum pyrexia. These must be recognized and managed promptly.

REFERENCES

1. Murphy KW. Reducing the complications of cesarean section. In Bonnar J.(ed). RA in Obstet Gynecol, Vol 20, Churchilll Livingstone, Edinburgh, 141–152, 1998.
2. Hema KR, Johonson R. Techniques for performing cesarean section. Best Pract Res clin Obstet Gynecol, 15(1);17–47, 2001.

16

Puerperal Pyrexia

Maitri C Shah, Saloni Prajapati

DEFINITION

Puerperal pyrexia is defined in the International Classification of Diseases (ICD-10), as a "temperature rise above 38.0°C (100.4°F) maintained over 24 hours or recurring during the period from the end of the first to the end of the tenth day after childbirth or abortion". While puerperal infection is most commonly encountered within the first 2 weeks after delivery, the definition extends to 42 days postpartum.[1]

CAUSES

Puerperal pyrexia encompasses all cases of significant pyrexia in the puerperium and includes not only infections due to puerperal sepsis, but also all extra-genital infections and incidental infections.[2,3] These can be broadly divided into the following groups:

1. Infections of the genito-urinary systems related to labor, delivery and the puerperium which include infection of vaginal/cervical laceration or episiotomy which can be either localized or has spread to the underlying soft tissue.
   - It may be caused by *E. coli*, other anaerobes, Group A Streptococcus, Staphylococcus spp. and *Clostridium welchii*.
2. Infections related to the uterus and its associated structures which includes postoperative infection following cesarean section.
   - Anaerobic conditions like surgical trauma, sutures, devitalized tissue and blood and serum facilitate bacterial proliferation and clinical infection.
3. Infections related to the urinary tract
   - 95% of these are caused by *Escherichia coli*, Proteus spp. and Klebsiella spp.
4. Infections specifically related to the birth process but not of the genito-urinary systems. These include:
   - Breast abscess (usually caused by Staphylococcus spp)
   - Deep vein thrombosis (DVT)
   - Incidental infections, e.g. malaria, respiratory tract infections

Some **non-infectious causes** of puerperal pyrexia include:
- Dehydration
- Tissue trauma
- Reaction to fetal proteins
- Breast engorgement.

Puerperal Sepsis and its Significance

It is defined as infection of the genital tract occurring at any time between the onset of rupture of membranes or labor, and the 42nd day postpartum in which two or more of the following are present:
- Pelvic pain
- Fever, i.e. oral temperature 38.5°C/101.3°F or higher on any occasion

- Abnormal vaginal discharge, e.g. presence of pus
- Abnormal smell/foul odour of discharge,
- Delay in the rate of reduction of the size of the uterus (involution) (< 2 cm/day during first 8 days).

Puerperal sepsis still continues to present a significant risk of obstetric morbidity and mortality to women in developing countries.[4] It is usually reported as the third or fourth leading cause of maternal death in this regions.[2] The infected mother in acute stage, suffers severe pain and is acutely ill very often ending in death. Often the recovery eventually result in infertility, chronic debilitation and life long suffering.[3]

RISK FACTORS FOR PUERPERAL PYREXIA[1,4,5]

Antepartum Factors

- Malnutrition and anemia
- HIV infection
- Preterm labor
- Preterm prelabor rupture of the membrane
- Chronic deliberating illness

Intrapartum Factors

- Repeated vaginal examination (>5)
- Prolonged labor (>12 hrs in active phase)
- Prolonged prelabor rupture of the membranes (>24 hrs)
- Dehydration and keto-acidosis during labor
- Traumatic operative delivery
- Hemorrhage-antepartum or postpartum
- Retained bits of the placental tissue or membranes
- Placental praevia–placental site lying close to the vagina
- Cesarean delivery

CLINICAL FEATURES

Clinical features vary depending on the source of infection and may include the following:[1]

- Fever and chills

- Flank pain, dysuria, and frequency of urinary tract infections
- Erythema and drainage from the surgical incision or episiotomy site, in cases of postsurgical wound infections (Figs 16.1 and 16.2)

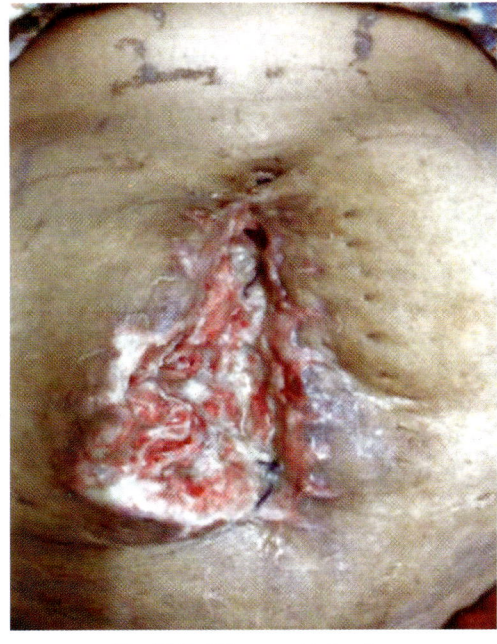

Fig. 16.1: CS wound infection

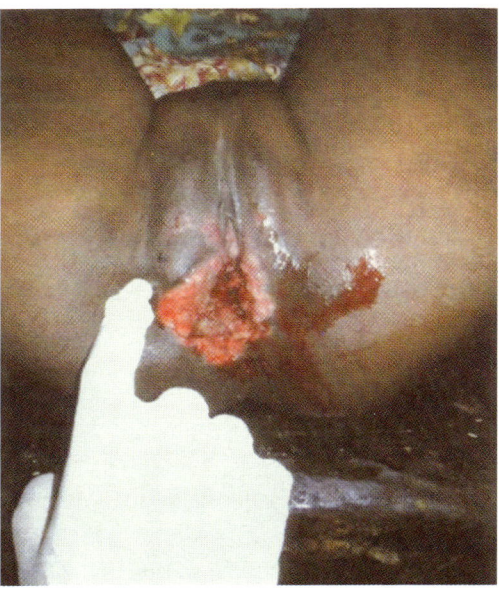

Fig. 16.2: Episio wound infection

- Respiratory symptoms, such as cough, pleuritic chest pain, or dyspnea, in cases of respiratory infection or septic pulmonary embolus
- Abdominal/pelvic pain and tenderness with delayed uterine involution
- Offensive vaginal discharge and heavy lochia
- Breast engorgement in cases of mastitis (Fig. 16.3)

MANAGEMENT OF PUERPERAL PYREXIA

1. History Taking

Antenatal history of anemia, antepartum hemorrhage, presence of septic foci in teeth, gums and tonsils, any debilitating diseases like heart disease, diabetes, tuberculosis and urinary tract infection or malaria should be inquired.

Intrapartun history regarding preterm labor, duration of rupture of membranes, number of internal examinations done, duration of labor, method of delivery, nature of intrauterine manipulation, if any.

Postnatal details of nature and frequency of fever, associated symptoms like burning micturition, breast engorgement, redness of breast, foul smelling vaginal discharge, lower abdominal pain, pain or swelling at stitch site etc. should be asked.

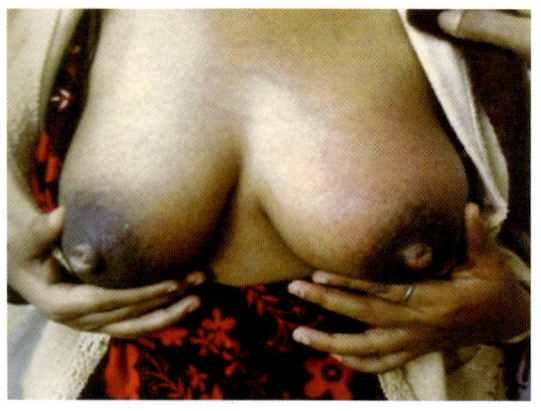

Fig. 16.3: Mastitis in left breast

2. Clinical Examination

- The focus of the physical examination should be on identifying the source of fever and infection.
- A complete physical examination, including pelvic and breast examinations shall be carried out.
- The speed of onset or deterioration in symptoms and signs is important.
- Clinical signs suggestive of sepsis include one or more of the following: pyrexia, hypothermia, tachycardia, tachypnoea, hypoxia, hypotension, oliguria, impaired consciousness and failure to respond to treatment.
- These signs, including pyrexia, may not always be present and are not necessarily related to the severity of sepsis.
- Life-threatening complications of severe sepsis include disseminated intravascular coagulation and adult respiratory distress syndrome
- In severe sepsis, there is evidence of organ dysfunction or hypoperfusion and hypotension is present.
- Septic shock is sepsis-induced hypotension, despite there being adequate arterial perfusion.[6]

Indications for hospital referral during puerperal period (Red flag signs and symptoms):[2]
Symptoms of sepsis in puerperium may be less distinctive than in the non-pregnant population and are not necessarily present in all cases; therefore, a high index of suspicion is necessary. Here, disease progression also may be rapid.

Any of the following signs during puerperium should prompt urgent referral for hospital assessment and, if the woman appears seriously unwell, by emergency ambulance.

- Pyrexia more than 38°C
- Sustained tachycardia more than 90 beats/minute

- Breathlessness (respiratory rate more than 20 breaths/minute; a serious symptom)
- Abdominal or chest pain
- Diarrhea and/or vomiting
- Uterine or renal angle pain and tenderness
- Woman is generally unwell or seems unduly anxious or distressed.

3. Investigations

- Blood cultures and other samples taken should be guided by clinical suspicion of focus of infection, such as throat swabs, mid-stream urine, high vaginal swab, placental swabs, sputum, cerebrospinal fluid, epidural site swab, cesarean section or episiotomy site wound swabs and expressed breast milk, and should ideally be obtained prior to starting antibiotic therapy as the results may become uninformative within a few hours of commencing antibiotics.
- Antibiotics should be given as soon as possible. Results of laboratory tests should be checked and recorded regularly and the medical microbiologist consulted to ensure specimens are processed appropriately and results communicated directly to the clinician at the earliest opportunity. Gram stain, culture results and sensitivities should be used to tailor antimicrobial therapy. If diarrhea is particularly offensive following antimicrobial therapy, a stool sample should be submitted for *C. difficile* toxin.

Baseline Investigations[3]

1. Complete blood count (CBC)
2. Bleeding time (BT) and clotting time (CT)
3. Blood for culture and antibiotic sensitivity
4. Urine routine and microscopic
5. Urine for culture and antibiotic sensitivity.
   Investigations to be carried out at higher center (specialised unit)[3]*

1. Full blood count (FBC)
2. Blood urea (BU)
3. Serum electrolytes (SE)
4. Liver function tests (LFT)
5. Blood for culture and antibiotic sensitivity
6. Coagulation profile.
7. Genital swabs (perineal, vaginal, high vaginal, endocervical swabs for culture and antibiotic sensitivity)
8. Ultrasound scan (USS) of pelvis
9. X-ray chest/abdomen (to detect perforations)

4. Management

- Treatment of puerperal infection usually begins with IV infusion of broad spectrum antibiotics and is continued for 48 hours after fever is resolved.
- IV access shall be established right at the primary centre and even primary course of antibiotics can be started even before getting any investigations done if needed.
- It always includes both supportive care and symptomatic treatment.
- Monitoring of these patients includes regular pulse and blood pressure recording (every 15 minutes), hourly monitoring of urine output through Foley catheter and central venous pressure (CVP) monitoring (where appropriate and when experienced staff is available).
- Surgery may be necessary to remove any remaining products of conception or to drain local lesions, such as an infected episiotomy (incision made during delivery) may need to be opened and drained.
- In the presence of thrombophlebitis, heparin therapy will be needed to provide anticoagulation.[3]

Choice of Antimicrobials[2,6,7]

- Antibiotic therapy should be guided by the Gram stain of any aspirate or biopsy;

* Intensive care unit (ICU); Care in collaboration with anesthesiologist is mandatory in severe sepsis/shock. Dedicated intensive care nurse per patient should be arranged whenever possible.

however, in practice the patient is usually so sick there is no time to wait, hence initial empirical prescribing of broad spectrum antibiotics is essential.

- Administration of intravenous broad-spectrum antibiotics within 1 hour of suspicion of severe sepsis, with or without septic shock, is recommended as part of the surviving sepsis resuscitation care bundle.
- If genital tract sepsis is suspected, prompt early treatment with a combination of high-dose broad spectrum intravenous antibiotics may be life saving.
- A combination of either piperacillin/tazobactam or a carbapenem plus clindamycin is a choice for severe sepsis.
- If the woman is or is highly likely to be MRSA-positive, vancomycin or teicoplanin may be added until sensitivity is known.
- Early presentation of sepsis (less than 12 hours post-birth) is more likely to be caused by streptococcal infection, particularly GAS, and severe continuous pain suggests necrotising fasciitis. The use of intravenous immunoglobulins in invasive streptococcal infections is still in the experimental stages.
- Breastfeeding is not contraindicated if the woman is clinically stable, but if there is clinical deterioration, then this issue must be addressed.
- However, breastfeeding limits the use of some antimicrobials; hence the advice of a consultant microbiologist should be sought at an early stage.
- Unless the mother is very ill, the newborn can stay with her. However, the precautions are necessary to prevent infection passing from the mother to the newborn.
- If the mother is very ill, a close relative may look after the baby at home.
- Careful observation of the newborn is essential to recognise early signs of infection.

Antimicrobial Choices and their Limitations[2]

Co-amoxiclav: Does not cover MRSA, pseudomonas or ESBL-producing organisms

Metronidazole: Only covers anaerobes

Clindamycin: Covers most streptococci and staphylococci, including many MRSA, and switches off exotoxin production with significantly decreased mortality not nephrotoxic

Piperacillin/tazobactam and carbapenems: Covers most organisms except MRSA and they are renal sparing (in contrast to aminoglycosides)

Piperacillin/tazobactam: Does not cover ESBL producers

Gentamicin (as a single dose of 3–5 mg/kg): Poses no problem in normal renal function but if doses are to be given regularly serum levels must be monitored.

Surgical Interventions[3]

- Infected episiotomies can be opened and allowed to drain. Abscesses and blood clots may require surgery.
- When multi-disciplinary approach is indicated the services of a surgeon, hematologist, pathologist and micro-biologist may be of paramount importance.
- Clot removal or by-pass. Sometimes, surgery is necessary to remove an acute clot blocking a pelvic vein or an abdominal vein. Procedures such as bypass/stent/filter may be necessary.
- Prompt and aggressive exploration and debridement of necrotic tissue are important.
- Hysterectomy is usually not needed; however, in severe cases involving large bacterial inocula, extensive tissue necrosis, or gangrene, hysterectomy and even removal of adenexal tissue might be indicated.

Prevention[1,7,8]

- Scrupulous attention to hygiene should be used during all examinations and use of instrumentation during and after labor. It is also necessary to reiterate the need for properly supervised labour and prompt use of oxytocics to prevent postpartum hemorrhage.
- Some centres advocate the use of prophylactic antibiotics during prolonged labor.
- Catheterisation should be avoided where possible.
- Perineal wounds should be cleaned and sutured as soon as possible after delivery.
- All blood losses and the completeness of the placenta should be recorded at all deliveries.
- Early mobilisation of delivered mothers will help to protect against venous thrombosis.
- New mothers should be helped to acquire the skills required for successful breast-feeding.
- Prophylactic antibiotics during operation reduces endometritis by 66–75% and also reduces rate of wound infection.
- Education, surveillance organisational change and quality improvement interventions should be introduced, confirming the need for a health systems approach to reduce maternal mortality especially in relation to sepsis.

REFERENCES

1. Standardised Maternal Guidelines on the Management of Puerperal Sepsis Developed for use in Health Facilities within the Western Cape. January 2008. Available at: http:/intrawp.pgwc.gov.za/health/cgac/default.asp

2. Bacterial Sepsis following Pregnancy. Royal College of Obstetricians & Gynecologists, Green–top Guideline No. 64b April 2012.

3. Dr DYK De Silva, Dr Athula Fernando et al. Management of Puerperal Sepsis. SLCOG National Guidelines.

4. Jeroen van Dillena, Joost Zwartb, Joke Schuttec and Jos van Roosmalen.Maternal sepsis: epidemiology, etiology and outcome. Current Opinion in Infectious Diseases 2010, 23: 249–254.

5. Dushyant Maharaj. Pyrexia: A Review. Part I. Obstetrical and Gynecological Survey. 62(6):393–9.

6. Palaniappan N, Menezes M,Willson P. Group A streptococcal puerperal sepsis: management and prevention. The Obstetrician & Gynecologist 2012(14)9–16.

7. Khaskheli MN, Baloch S, Sheeba A. Risk factors and complications of puerperal sepsis at a tertiary healthcare centre. Pak J Med Sci 2013;29(4):972–6.

8. Etim Inyang Ekanem, Efiok Eyo Efiok, Atim Edet Udoh, Etop Charles Anaikot. Trends in postpartum maternal morbidity in Ikot Ekpene a rural community in Southern Nigeria. Open Journal of Obstetrics and Gynecology, 2013, (3): 493–9.

Section
IV

Specific Diseases
in Pregnancy

17

Hepatitis in Pregnancy

Preeti Yogesh Bhandari

INTRODUCTION

There is a subset of liver diseases uniquely associated with pregnancy, whereas others are unrelated. The liver diseases unique to pregnancy include hyperemesis gravidarum, acute fatty liver of pregnancy, intrahepatic cholestasis of pregnancy, and HELLP syndrome. While the liver diseases incidental to pregnancy are viral hepatitis, liver cirrhosis, autoimmune hepatitis, hepatocellular carcinomas and the list is endless.

Pregnancy presents unique challenges in the diagnosis and management of liver diseases.

ANATOMICAL AND PHYSIOLOGICAL CHANGES IN LIVER DURING PREGNANCY

There is no change in the size of the liver in normal pregnant woman.

Pregnancy causes very few alterations in the results of standard liver tests. The aminotransferases (AST and ALT), g-glutamyltranspeptidase (GGTP), total bilirubin, and serum bile acid level remain within the normal range. Serum alkaline phosphatase levels almost double during normal pregnancy, mainly due to placental alkaline phosphatase. The alkaline phosphatase rises modestly in the third trimester.[1]

VIRAL HEPATITIS

Viral hepatitis is the inflammation of the liver due to a viral infection. It may present as an acute or chronic infection. The most common causes of viral hepatitis are hepatotropic viruses hepatitis A, B, C, D and E. Cytomegalovirus, Epstein-Barr virus and yellow fever are the other viruses known to cause viral hepatitis. The clinical course of most of the viral hepatitis infections is unaffected by pregnancy except hepatitis E and disseminated herpes simplex hepatitis.

Hepatitis A

Incidence of HAV in pregnancy is 1 in 1000.[2] The causative agent hepatitis A RNA virus is spread via the fecal-oral route and is more prevalent in low socioeconomic areas where a lack of adequate sanitation and poor hygienic practices facilitate spread of the infection.

Hepatitis A virus (HAV) infection usually results in an acute, self-limited illness and only rarely leads to fulminant hepatic failure.[3] Fulminant hepatic failure occurs more commonly in patients with underlying liver disease, particularly chronic hepatitis C virus (HCV) infection.

Laboratory abnormalities may include marked elevations of serum aminotransferases (usually >1000 IU/dL), serum total and direct bilirubin, and alkaline phosphatase.[4] Serum bilirubin levels above 10 mg/dL are common. Other laboratory abnormalities include nonspecific elevations of acute phase reactants, elevated erythrocyte sedimentation rate, and increased immunoglobulins.

The diagnosis of acute hepatitis A virus (HAV) infection is made by the detection of anti-HAV antibodies in a patient with the typical clinical presentation. Serum IgM anti-HAV is the gold standard for the detection of acute illness.[5]

Implications specific to pregnant women and neonates: The clinical course of hepatitis A is similar to that in non-pregnant patients. Nausea and vomiting may be confused with symptoms of early pregnancy. Preterm labor can occur if infection occurs in the third trimester of pregnancy. Fetal transmission is rare but may occur if delivery takes place during incubation period because of viral shedding and contamination during vaginal delivery.

IgG antibodies to HAV are positively transmitted to the newborn and provide protection to the infant in initial months of life. Breastfeeding is not contraindicated.

HAV vaccination may be given during pregnancy to persons at high risk for acquiring infection,[6] e.g. travelers to high risk areas, patients with chronic liver disease and patients with clotting factor disorders.

Either inactivated virus vaccine or recombinant vaccine is available and safe in pregnancy. Protection of vaccine lasts up to 12 months after single dose and up to 20 years after second dose.

Newborn of mother with hepatitis A in the third trimester should be given passive immunoprophylaxis with immunoglobulin within 48 hours of birth. The dose is 0.02 ml/kg body weight.

Hepatitis E

Hepatitis E virus (HEV) is an enterically-transmitted acute viral hepatitis. Infection with this virus was first documented in 1955 during an outbreak in New Delhi, India.[7]

The epidemiology of hepatitis E virus (HEV), previously known as waterborne or enterically transmitted non-A, non-B hepatitis, is similar to that of hepatitis A virus. However, HAV is more readily transmitted, causes more infections, and has a wider distribution worldwide.

The highest incidence of HEV infection is in Asia, Africa, Middle East, and Central America. It is the most common form of hepatitis which can occur in an epidemic form. In the largest reported outbreak, over 100,000 individuals were infected in the Xinjiang region of China between 1986 and 1988.[8]

High attack rates are found in adults between 15 and 40 years of age. Secondary attack rates from person-to-person transmission in susceptible households are uncommon but have been documented. HEV is spread by fecally contaminated water in endemic areas.

HEV generally causes a self-limited acute infection, although fulminant hepatitis can develop. Chronic hepatitis does not develop after acute HEV infection, except in the transplant setting and possibly in other settings of immunosuppression.

The incubation period of HEV infection ranges from 15 to 60 days. The clinical signs and symptoms in patients with typical HEV infection are similar to those seen with other forms of acute viral hepatitis, although disease appears to be relatively severe compared with hepatitis A.

Laboratory findings include elevated serum concentrations of bilirubin, alanine aminotransferase (ALT), and aspartate aminotransferase (AST). Resolution of the abnormal biochemical tests generally occurs within one to six weeks after the onset of the illness.

The diagnosis of HEV is based upon the detection of HEV in serum or stool by polymerase chain reaction (PCR) or by the detection of IgM antibodies to HEV. Serological and nucleic acid tests (qualitative and quantitative HEV RNA) currently represent the gold-standard for testing for HEV.

Implications specific to pregnant women and neonates: There is a little information regarding the vertical transmission of HEV from infected mothers to their infants.

For reasons that are not understood, fulminant hepatic failure occurs more frequently during pregnancy, resulting in an inordinately high mortality rate of 15 to 25 percent, primarily in women in the third trimester.[9] A contributing factor may be that pregnancy predisposes to increased viral replication.[9] Pregnant women with jaundice and acute viral hepatitis caused by HEV infection appear to have worse obstetric and fetal outcomes compared to pregnant women with jaundice and acute viral hepatitis due to other causes.

Treatment of HEV infection remains supportive, as the disease appears to be self-limiting in non-immunocompromised patients.

Liver transplantation may be required in severe hepatitis with liver failure.

Hepatitis B

Hepatitis B (HBV) is caused by a double stranded DNA virus with an incubation period of 45–160 days. Modes of transmission are parenteral, sexual contact, mucosal exposure to blood and infected body fluids and vertical. Among regular sexual contacts of HBV infected persons, 25% become seropositive.[10] It is an occupational risk for healthcare workers and nurses. The risk of transmission with percutaneous exposure is 6 to 30%. Body fluids and blood of the patient are highly infectious and very small amount of blood is required for transmission.

Hepatitis B during pregnancy presents with unique management issues for both the mother and fetus. These include the effects of HBV on maternal and fetal health, the effects of pregnancy on the course of HBV infection, treatment of HBV during pregnancy, and prevention of perinatal transmission. Vertical transmission is responsible for approximately one-half of chronic infection worldwide.

The risk of developing chronic HBV infection is inversely proportional to the age at time of exposure. The risk is as high as 90 percent in those exposed at birth, while the risk is much lower (about 20 to 30 percent) in those exposed during childhood. Identification of at-risk mothers permits prophylaxis against transmission, which can reduce transmission rates from 90 percent to as low as 5 to 10 percent.[11]

Implications of HBV infection for the mother

Acute HBV infection during pregnancy is usually not severe and is not associated with increased mortality or teratogenicity.[12] Thus, infection during gestation should not prompt consideration of termination of the pregnancy. Acute HBV occurring early in the pregnancy has been associated with a 10 percent perinatal transmission rate. Transmission rates significantly increase if acute infection occurs at or near the time of delivery, with rates reported as high as 60 percent.[12]

Treatment of acute infection during pregnancy is mainly supportive. Liver biochemical tests and prothrombin time should be monitored. Antiviral therapy is usually unnecessary, except in women who have acute liver failure or protracted severe hepatitis. Lamivudine (100 mg daily) is a reasonable option since it has been used safely during pregnancy and the anticipated duration of treatment is short.

Chronic HBV

Pregnancy is generally well-tolerated by women with chronic hepatitis B infection who do not have advanced liver disease. Occasional patients develop a hepatitis flare, therefore HBsAg-positive mothers should be monitored closely.

Implications of HBV infection for the infant: Maternal-infant transmission can occur in utero, at birth, or after birth. Most infections occur at birth when maternal secretions in the birth canal come in contact with the infant's mucosal membranes.

The most important risk factor for transmission despite proper administration of prophylaxis appears to be high maternal HBV viral load. Transplacental transmission and transmission due to obstetrical procedures are less frequent causes, while breastfeeding does not appear to pose a substantial risk. The benefit of cesarean delivery in protecting against transmission has not been clearly established. The obstetrical approach should not be influenced by the HBV status of the mother.[13]

Children born to HBeAg-positive mothers remain at risk for HBV infection, even if they receive vaccination and HBIG (approximately 9 percent in one large cohort study).[14]

Maternal serum HBV DNA levels correlate with the risk of transmission. Vertical transmission of hepatitis B occurs in 9 to 39 percent of infants of highly viremic mothers despite postnatal vaccination.[15]

Transmission following amniocentesis has been described, but the risk appears to be low, particularly in mothers who are HBeAg negative and when the procedure is done using a 22-gauge needle under continuous guidance.[16] The effect of other invasive procedures during pregnancy (e.g. chorionic villus sampling, cordocentesis, fetal surgery) on the risk of transmission is unknown.

Breastfeeding does not appear to increase the risk of transmission. Infants who received HBIG and the first dose of vaccine at birth can be breastfed as long as they complete the course of vaccination, but carrier mothers should not participate in donating breast milk. Mothers with chronic hepatitis B who are breastfeeding should also exercise care to prevent bleeding from cracked nipples.

Testing for HBsAg should be performed on all women at the first prenatal visit and repeated late in pregnancy in those at high risk for HBV infection.

In addition to standard passive-active immunization, antiviral therapy should be offered to mothers with high HBV DNA levels since it can further reduce the risk of perinatal transmission. However, more data are needed to clarify the HBV DNA cutoff for recommending antiviral therapy to pregnant chronic HBV women.

Various factors need to be considered when deciding on antiviral therapy during pregnancy including the indications, anticipated duration of therapy, potential adverse effects to the fetus, efficacy, and the risk of development of drug resistance. The safety of medication exposure in the fetus needs to be weighed against the risk of stopping or changing therapy for the mother.

There are generally two indications for antiviral therapy during pregnancy:

- Treatment of chronic disease in the mother
- Treatment to decrease the risk of perinatal transmission

Based upon current data, lamivudine and tenofovir are preferred if antiviral therapy is contemplated in pregnant women. Tenofovir is a better choice in women who will receive long-term treatment because of a low risk of resistance.

When antiviral therapy should be discontinued, postpartum has not been determined. Many experts would stop treatment 4 to 12 weeks after delivery if the sole purpose of antiviral therapy is to decrease the risk of maternal-infant transmission. Close monitoring is necessary after treatment is discontinued because of the possibility of a developing a hepatitis flare.

Hepatitis C

HCV is a partially double-stranded RNA virus. Infection with this virus is a major cause of chronic hepatitis, cirrhosis, and hepatocellular carcinoma (HCC) around the world. HCV disease has a slow onset with symptoms in about 25% of patients. Approximately 75% of patients are chronically infected and may not be aware of their infection, because they are not clinically ill.

Implications specific to pregnant women and neonates: In the pregnant population, the prevalence of HCV is estimated to be about 1%.[17]

Transfer of HCV infection in pregnancy occurs as a result of vertical or horizontal transfer. The rate of mother-to-infant transmission is 4–7% per pregnancy among women with detectable viremia.[17]

Vertical perinatal transmission occurs in women who are HCV-RNA positive at the time of delivery and appears to be highly dependent on viral load and HIV status, which are independent of each other.[18] High HCV viral loads of more than 100,000 copies/mL are associated with an increased risk of vertical transmission.

Evidence from large multicenter trials does not support elective cesarean delivery for prevention of vertical HCV transmission.[19]

Autoimmune Hepatitis

This is a progressive liver disease mainly affecting females. Remission or flare ups can occur in pregnancy and labor. There is increased incidence of preterm labor, low birth weight and fetal loss. Immunosupressive therapy should be continued during pregnancy. Diagnosis is by detection of anti-nuclear antibody, anti-smooth muscle antibody, anti-liver kidney microsomal antibody. Treatment options for flare of autoimmune hepatitis include steroids and azathioprine.

Evidence based recommendations by American College of Obstetricians and Gynecologists (ACOG) executive board on hepatitis in pregnancy:[20]

Level A

- Routine prenatal screening of all pregnant women by hepatitis B surface antigen (HBsAg) testing is recommended.
- Newborns born to hepatitis B carriers should receive combined immunoprophylaxis consisting of hepatitis B immune globulin (HBIG) and hepatitis B vaccine within 12 hours of birth.
- Hepatitis B infection is a preventable disease, and all at risk individuals, particularly healthcare workers, should be vaccinated. All infants, should receive the hepatitis B vaccine series as part of the childhood recommended immunization schedule.
- Breastfeeding is not contraindicated in women with hepatitis A virus infection with appropriate hygienic precautions, in those chronically infected with hepatitis B if the infant receives HBIG passive prophylaxis and vaccine active prophylaxis or in women with hepatitis C virus infection.

Level B

- Routine prenatal HCV screening is not recommended; however, women with significant risk factors for infection should be offered antibody screening.
- Route of delivery has not been shown to influence the risk of vertical HCV transmission, and cesarean delivery should be reserved for obstetric indications in women with HCV infection.

Level C

- The risk of transmission of hepatitis B associated with amniocentesis is low.
- Susceptible pregnant women who are at risk for hepatitis B infections should be specifically targeted for vaccination.

REFERENCES

1. Bacq Y, Zarka O, Brechot J-F, et al. Liver function tests in normal pregnancy: A prospective study of 103 pregnant women and 103 matched controls. Hepatology 1996;23:1030–4.
2. Leikin E, Lysikiewicz A, Garry D, Tejani N. Intrauterine transmission of hepatitis A virus. ObstetGynecol 1996; 88:690–91.
3. Taylor RM, Davern T, Munoz S, et al. Fulminant hepatitis A virus infection in the United States: Incidence, prognosis, and outcomes. Hepatology 2006; 44:1589.
4. Tong MJ, el-Farra NS, Grew MI. Clinical manifestations of hepatitis A: recent experience in a community teaching hospital. J Infect Dis 1995; 171 Suppl 1:S15.
5. Centers for Disease Control and Prevention (CDC). Positive test results for acute hepatitis A virus infection among persons with no recent history of acute hepatitis—United States, 2002–2004. MMWR Morb Mortal Wkly Rep 2005; 54:453.
6. Prevention of hepatitis A through active or passive immunization: Recommendations of the Advisory Committee on Immunization Practices (ACIP). MMWR Recomm Rep 1996;45:1–30.
7. Gupta DN, Smetana HF. The histopathology of viral hepatitis as seen in the Delhi epidemic (1955–56). Indian J Med Res 1957; 45:101.
8. Zhuang H. Hepatitis E and strategies for its control. Viral Hepatitis in China: Problems and Control Strategies. MonogrVirol 1992; 19:126
9. Kar P, Jilani N, Husain SA, et al. Does hepatitis E viral load and genotypes influence the final outcome of acute liver failure during pregnancy? Am J Gastroenterol 2008; 103:2495.
10. ASRM Practice Committee. Hepatitis and reproduction. FertilSteril 2008.
11. Stevens CE, Beasley RP, Tsui J, Lee WC. Vertical transmission of hepatitis B antigen in Taiwan. N Engl J Med 1975; 292:771.
12. Jonas MM. Hepatitis B and pregnancy: An underestimated issue. Liver Int 2009; 29 Suppl 1:133.
13. Yang J, Zeng XM, Men YL, Zhao LS. Elective caesarean section versus vaginal delivery for preventing mother to child transmission of hepatitis B virus—a systematic review. Virol J 2008; 5:100.
14. Chen HL, Lin LH, Hu FC, et al. Effects of maternal screening and universal immunization to prevent mother-to-infant transmission of HBV. Gastroenterology 2012; 142:773.
15. Pan C, Han GR, Zhao W, et al. Virologic factors associated with failure to passive-active immunoprophylaxis in infants with HBsAg-positive at birth. Hepatology 2011; 54:878A.
16. López M, Coll O. Chronic viral infections and invasive procedures: Risk of vertical transmission and current recommendations. Fetal DiagnTher 2010; 28:1.
17. Berger A. Science commentary. Behaviour Of hepatitis C virus. BMJ. 1998 Aug 15. 317(7156): 437A.
18. Lin HH, Kao JH, Hsu HY, Ni YH, Yeh SH, Hwang LH. Possible role of high-titer maternal viremia in perinatal transmission of hepatitis C virus. J Infect Dis. 1994 Mar. 169(3):638–41.
19. Pembrey L, Newell ML, Tovo PA. The management of HCV infected pregnant women and their children European paediatric HCV network. J Hepatol. 2005 Sep. 43(3):515–25.
20. American College of Obstetricians and Gynecologists (ACOG). Viral hepatitis in pregnancy. Washington (DC): ACOG practice bulletin no. 86; 2007 Oct 15p.

18

The Diagnosis and Treatment of Malaria in Pregnancy

Khushboo Bagdi, Reena Wani

INTRODUCTION AND LIFE CYCLE

Malaria is the most important parasitic infection in the tropical areas. Its name is derived from the belief of the ancient Romans that *malaria* was due to the bad air of the marshes surrounding Rome. Malaria in pregnancy is detrimental to the woman and her fetus. The protozoan parasites *P. falciparum*, *P. vivax*, *P. malariae* and *P. ovale* (extremely rarely *P. knowlesi*), are transmitted by the bite of a sporozoite-bearing female anopheline mosquito. After a period of pre-erythrocytic development in the liver, the blood stage infection begins. Parasitic invasion of the erythrocyte consumes haemoglobin and alters the red cell membrane. This allows *P. falciparum* infected erythrocytes to cytoadhere inside the small blood vessels which interfere with microcirculatory flow and metabolism of vital organs.

The hallmark of falciparum malaria in pregnancy is parasites sequestered in the placenta. Sequestration is not known to occur by other parasites. In pregnancy, the adverse effects of malaria infection result from:

- *The systemic infection*: Maternal and fetal mortality, miscarriage, stillbirth and premature birth
- *The parasitisation itself*: Fetal growth restriction and low birth weight, maternal and fetal anemia, interaction with HIV, susceptibility of the infant to malaria.

P. falciparum causes greater morbidity and mortality than non-falciparum infections but there is mounting evidence that *P. vivax* is not as benign as had been previously thought.

DIAGNOSIS OF MALARIA IN PREGNANCY

Suspicion of malaria requires prompt confirmation by malaria blood film, as there are no clinical algorithms that permit accurate diagnosis by signs and symptoms. In its early stages, the symptoms and signs of malaria can mimic influenza/viral infections.

Symptoms

Fever/chills/sweats, headache, muscle pain, nausea, vomiting, diarrhea, cough, general malaise

Signs

Jaundice, elevated temperature, perspiration, pallor, splenomegaly, respiratory distress.

How should malaria in pregnancy be diagnosed?

The diagnosis of malaria relies on microscopic examination (the current gold standard) of thick and thin blood films for parasites or the use of rapid diagnostic tests which detect specific parasite antigen or enzyme (RMAT or Rapid Malaria Antigen Detection Tests). Rapid detection tests may miss low parasitaemia, which is more likely in pregnant women, and are relatively insensitive in *P. vivax* malaria.[1] A positive rapid diagnostic test should be followed by microscopy to quantify the number of infected red blood cells (parasitaemia) and to confirm the species and the stage of parasites. In a febrile patient, 3 negative malaria smears 12–24 hours apart rules out the diagnosis of malaria.

A study by us comparing use of diagnostic tests in pregnant women with fever found that despite all its advantages and usefulness in field situations and low-resource settings, RMAT will not be able to replace microscopy. Microscopy is still more flexible and offers immense advantage of providing species diagnosis and exact parasite densities. RMAT can be used at times where there is urgent need of diagnosis to prevent mortality and morbidity.[2]

PS for MP is gold standard for diagnosis and gives additional information regarding type of parasite and density, however, it requires expertise. RMAT is available, easy to perform and it is recommended that all RMAT are followed-up with microscopy to confirm the results and if positive, to quantify the proportion of red blood cells that are infected.[2]

Other important prognostic factors that should be reported on a peripheral blood smear result are:

- The presence and count of mature trophozoites and schizonts of *P. falciparum*
- Finding malaria pigment in more than 5% of the polymorphonuclear leucocytes in the peripheral blood film.

Is the severity of malaria a useful aid in managing the infection?

Clinical and laboratory findings of **severe/ complicated malaria** in adults are as follows.

Clinical Manifestations

- Prostration
- Impaired consciousness

- Respiratory distress (acidotic breathing, acute respiratory distress syndrome, pulmonary edema*)
- Multiple convulsions
- Circulatory collapse, shock (blood pressure < 90/60 mmHg)
- Abnormal bleeding, disseminated intra-vascular coagulopathy
- Jaundice
- Hemoglobinuria (without G6PD deficiency)

Laboratory Tests

- Severe anemia (hemoglobin < 8.0 g/dl)
- Thrombocytopenia
- Hypoglycemia (< 2.2 mmol/l)*
- Acidosis (pH < 7.3)
- Renal impairment (oliguria < 0.4 ml/kg body weight/hour or creatinine > 265 µmol/l)
- Hyperlactatemia
- Hyperparasitemia (>2% parasitised red blood cells)
- Algid malaria—Gram-negative septicaemia*
- Lumbar puncture to exclude meningitis.

The severity of malaria determines the treatment and predicts the case fatality rate. In uncomplicated malaria, fatality rates are low: approximately 0.1% for *P. falciparum*. In severe malaria, particularly in pregnancy, fatality rates are high (15–20% in nonpregnant women compared with 50% in pregnancy). Brabin estimated mortality to be 2–10 times higher in pregnant women than in non-pregnant women in endemic areas.[3] The non-falciparum species are rarely fatal but caution should still be observed.

How is malaria infection treated during pregnancy?

Treat malaria in pregnancy as an emergency.

Seek advice from infectious diseases specialists, especially for severe and recurrent cases.

*Common features in pregnant women with severe or complicated malaria.

Drug Treatment

Our vector-borne disease control program (NVBDCP 2013) has given guidelines, these have been discussed in the preceding chapter on Fever in Monsoon. International guidelines in pregnant women are essentially similar as given below: UK treatment guidelines in pregnancy.[4]

Severe or Complicated Malaria

- Artesunate IV 2.4 mg/kg at 0, 12 and 24 hours, then daily thereafter. When the patient is well enough to take oral medication she can be switched to oral artesunate 2 mg/kg (or IM artesunate 2.4 mg/kg) once daily, plus clindamycin. If oral artesunate is not available, use a 3-day course of atovaquone-proguanil or a 7-day course of quinine and clindamycin at 450 mg 3 times a day for 7 days.
- Alternatively, quinine IV 20 mg/kg loading dose (no loading dose if patient already taking quinine or mefloquine) in 5% dextrose over 4 hours and then 10 mg/kg IV over 4 hours every 8 hours plus clindamycin IV 450 mg every 8 hours (max. dose quinine 1.4 g). When the patient is well enough to take oral medication she can be switched to oral quinine 600 mg 3 times a day to complete 5–7 days and oral clindamycin 450 mg 3 times a day 7 days (an alternative rapid quinine-loading regimen is 7 mg/kg quinine dihyrochloride IV over 30 minutes using an infusion pump followed by 10 mg/kg over 4 hours).

Note: Quinine dosing should be reduced to 12-hourly dosing if IV therapy extends more than 48 hours or if the patient has renal or hepatic dysfunction. Quinine is associated with severe and recurrent hypoglycemia in late pregnancy.

Uncomplicated Malaria by *P. Falciparum*

- Oral quinine 600 mg 8 hourly and oral clindamycin 450 mg 8 hourly for 7 days (can be given together)
- Alternativey, atovaquone-proguanil 4 standard tablets daily for 3 days.

Vomiting but No Signs of Severe Complicated Malaria

Quinine 10 mg/kg dose IV in 5% dextrose over 4 hours every 8 hours plus IV clindamycin 450 mg every 8 hours. When the patient is well enough to take oral medication she can be switched to oral quinine 600 mg 3 times a day to complete 5–7 days and oral clindamycin can if needed be switched to 450 mg 3 times a day 7 days.

Non-falciparum Malaria

P. vivax, P. ovale, P. malariae: Oral chloroquine (base) 600 mg followed by 300 mg 68 hours later. Then 300 mg on day 2 and again on day 3.

Resistant P. vivax: As for uncomplicated malaria *P. falciparum.*

Preventing relapse during pregnancy: Chloroquine oral 300 mg weekly until delivery.

Preventing relapse after delivery: Postpone until 3 months after delivery and G6PD testing.

P. ovale: Oral primaquine 15 mg single daily dose for 14 days.

P. vivax: Oral primaquine 30 mg single daily dose for 14 days.

G6PD (mild) for P. vivax or P. ovale: Primaquine oral 45–60 mg once a week for 8 weeks.

Where should treatment of uncomplicated malaria infection take place?

It is advisable to hospitalise all pregnant women with *P. falciparum*, as the clinical condition can deteriorate rapidly.[4] Quinine has significant adverse effects, principally cinchonism, which includes tinnitus, headache, nausea, diarrhoea, altered auditory acuity and blurred vision which can lead to non-compliance.[5] For this reason, hospitalisation can be useful. While non-falciparum malaria can be managed on an outpatient basis, admission ensures compliance.

What happens if the patient vomits?

Vomiting is a symptom of malaria and a known adverse effect of quinine. If the patient vomits, use an antiemetic. Metoclopramide is considered safe, even in the first trimester.[6] After the antiemetic has had time to take effect, repeat the dose. Repeat vomiting after antiemetic is an indication for parenteral therapy.

What other medication should be provided alongside treatment of uncomplicated malaria infection?

The fever of malaria has been associated with premature labor [7] and fetal distress.[8] Prompt treatment with antipyretics is fundamental to the treatment of fever.

Mild and moderate malaria-associated anaemia is treated with ferrous sulphate and folic acid at the usual doses.

Does pregnancy affect the efficacy of malaria treatments?

Treatments in pregnancy may have lower efficacy than in non-pregnant patients but this apparent effect could result from lowered concentrations of antimalarials in pregnancy.

Malaria in pregnancy is unique and the ability of P. falciparum to sequester in the placenta challenges the normal way antimalarial drug efficacy is assessed. Polymerase chain reaction (PCR) confirmed prolonged submicroscopic carriage with subsequent recurrence has been reported in pregnant women for months following drug treatment for uncomplicated P. falciparum. Most recurrence is around day 28–42 but late-reported recurrence, so far unique to pregnancy, has been reported to occur at 85 days with quinine, 98 days with artesunate,

63 days with artemether-lumefantrine and 121 days with mefloquine. Weekly screening by blood film until delivery detects malaria before becoming symptomatic.

How should recurrence be treated?

The treatment efficacy of antimalarials for recurrent malaria in pregnancy is not known. The cure rates for uncomplicated malaria with quinine fell from 77.0% to 61.0% (P = 0.03) and for mefloquine from 72.0% to 62.5% (P> 0.05) when these drugs were used to treat primary and recurrent infections.[9] The alternative regimen for recurrent malaria at that time (1995–1997) was artesunate monotherapy, which had a cure rate of 84%. A highly effective 7-day treatment has more chance of curing the patient.

Atovaquone-proguanil-artesunate[10] and dihydroartemisinin-piperaquine[11] have been used in pregnant women with multiple recurrent infections with good effect. The WHO recommended regimen of 7 days of artesunate (2 mg/kg/day or 100 mg daily for 7 days) and clindamycin (450 mg three times daily for 7 days) could be given.

How are pregnancy-related complications of severe malaria managed?

Severe malaria in pregnancy is a medical emergency and women should be treated in a high-dependency or ICU, according to their condition. While hypoglycaemia, pulmonary edema, severe anemia and secondary bacterial infection can occur in severe malaria in non-pregnant patients, they are more common and severe in pregnant women.[4]

Hypoglycemia is commonly asymptomatic, although it may be associated with fetal bradycardia and other signs of fetal distress. In the most severely ill women, it is associated with lactic acidosis and high mortality. The hypoglycemia of quinine is caused by hyperinsulinemia and may be profound, recurrent and intractable in pregnancy.[8] It may present late in the disease when the patient appears to be recovering.[8]

Pulmonary edema may be present on admission or may develop suddenly. It may develop immediately after childbirth. Pulmonary edema is a grave complication, with a high mortality of over 50%.[12] The first indication of impending pulmonary edema is an increase in the respiratory rate, which precedes the development of other chest signs. Ensure that the pulmonary edema has not resulted from iatrogenic fluid overload and monitor the central venous pressure and urine output. In some women, ARDS can occur in addition to the pulmonary edema.

Severe anemia is associated with maternal morbidity, an increased risk of postpartum hemorrhage and perinatal mortality. Women who go into labor when severely anemic or fluid-overloaded may develop acute pulmonary edema after separation of the placenta. Monitor hemoglobin and transfuse as necessary. Exchange transfusion may be considered but there is no clear evidence base.

Secondary bacterial infection, principally Gram-negative septicaemia, has been reported.[13] Blood cultures should be taken if the patient shows signs of shock or fever returns after apparent fever clearance, Broad-spectrum antibiotics (such as ceftriaxone) should be started immediately. Once the results of blood culture are available, give the appropriate antibiotic.

Obstetric Management Specific to Malaria Infection in Pregnancy

Common Obstetric Problems with Acute Symptomatic Malaria

- Preterm labour, fetal growth restriction and fetal heart rate abnormalities can occur in malaria in pregnancy.
- In severe malaria, cardiotocograph monitoring may reveal fetal tachycardia, bradycardia or late decelerations in relation to uterine contractions, indicating fetal distress; particularly in the presence of fever.[7]

  – Paracetamol 1 g every 4–6 hours (to a maximum of 4 g/day) is safe and effective.
- Maternal hypoglycaemia should be excluded as the cause of fetal distress.
- Tocolytic therapy and prophylactic steroid therapy at the usual obstetric doses should be considered if there are no contra-indications.
- In severe malaria complicated by fetal compromise, a multidisciplinary team approach (intensive care specialist, infectious disease specialist, obstetrician, neonatologist) is required to plan optimal management.

Abnormalities in fetal and placental circulation have been noted on **Doppler studies**. In one study, 23 women with acute malaria reported that the umbilical artery resistance index increased by 5 to 20% (P < 0.05), with evidence of cerebral redistribution.[14]

Most epidemiologic studies conducted in malaria-endemic countries have found that primigravidae are more susceptible to malaria than multigravidae. In an area of moderate malaria transmission in Africa, women of all parities had substantially increased risk of low birthweight and severe anemia as a result of malaria infection in pregnancy. The risk of low birthweight is likely to be particularly high in areas with a high prevalence of severe anemia.[15]

In the second observational study in Kenya, malaria infection at 32–35 weeks of gestation was associated with abnormal uterine artery flow velocity waveforms on the day of blood testing (RR 2.11; 95% CI 1.24–3.59; P= 0.006).[14] Uncomplicated malaria in pregnancy is not a reason for **induction of labor**. Instrumental birth in the second stage of labor in the presence of maternal or fetal distress is indicated, if there are no contraindications. In severe malaria, the role of early cesarean section for the viable fetus is unproven.

Coagulation Disorders

- There is usually no need for pregnant women with malaria infection to receive **thromboprophylaxis**.
- Acute malaria causes **thrombocytopenia** and, in severe malaria, can cause DIC. Thrombocytopenia recovers with treatment: 90% by day 7 and 100% by day 14, irrespective of the type of antimalarial treatment.
- Studies show **postpartum hemorrhage** to be higher in malarious areas compared with non-malarious areas of Papua New Guinea.[16]

What antenatal care after recovery from an episode of malaria in pregnancy is advised?

Regular antenatal care, including assessment of maternal hemoglobin, platelets, glucose and fetal growth scans, is advised following recovery from an episode of malaria in pregnancy. Regular fetal growth assessment is advised and, if growth restriction is identified, routine obstetric management for this condition applies investigation.

Effective antimalarial treatment which clears the placenta of parasites is the most important step in preventing this complication followed by prophylaxis to prevent relapse, such as weekly chloroquine for *P. vivax*. The chances of recurrence are low when a woman has completed an effective course of antimalarials. Nevertheless, it is useful for women to be aware that malaria can recur (more likely with *P. vivax* or *P. ovale*). Should symptoms return, prompt screening by malaria blood film, is essential.

Plasmodium falciparum—infected erythrocytes frequently sequester in the intervillous space of the placenta and cause pathologic alterations. Placental malaria has been associated with a significant decrease in infant birth weight, especially in primigravidea. It has also been identified as a risk factor for low birth weight (LBW) babies.[17]

The post-malaria treatment course for women treated for malaria can be complicated by anemia, which will be detected in routine antenatal screening. There are malaria-endemic countries where the risk of pre-eclampsia is increased significantly in women with placental malaria.

Congenital Malaria

Antimalarial drugs can clear peripheral parasitaemia more quickly than from the placenta. Maternal malaria close to delivery can result in congenital malaria, which can cause significant mortality. Congenital malaria may present in the first weeks to months of life.

A negative placental blood film at delivery in a woman who has had malaria in pregnancy eliminates the risk of congenital malaria significantly. Placenta- and cord-positive blood films result in a higher chance of congenital malaria than placenta-positive, cord-negative blood films. Send the placenta for histopathology, as it is more sensitive than microscopy for detection of placental parasites.[18]

What is the risk of vertical transmission of malaria infection to the baby?

Vertical transmission to the fetus can occur particularly when there is infection at the time of birth and the placenta and cord are blood film positive for malaria. Infection of the newborn can occur despite appropriate treatment in the mother during pregnancy.

All neonates whose mothers developed malaria in pregnancy should be screened for malaria with standard microscopy of thick and thin blood films at birth and weekly blood films for 28 days, if the placenta is positive for parasites.

REFERENCES

1. Ashley EA, Touabi M, Ahrer M, Hutagalung R, Htun K, Luchavez J, et al. Evaluation of three parasite lactate dehydrogenase-based rapid

diagnostic tests for the diagnosis of falciparum and vivax malaria. Malar J 2009;8: 241.

2. Diagnosis of Malaria in pregnancy: Field situation and use of rapid tests. Reena Wani, Anjali Swami, Namrata Rajput, Jayanthi Shastri. The Indian Practitioner, Vol. 67 No. 1, Jan 2014, p23–27.

3. Brabin BJ. An analysis of malaria in pregnancy in Africa. Bull World Health Organ1983;61:1005–16.

4. Lalloo DG, Shingadia D, Pasvol G, Chiodini PL, Whitty CJ, Beeching NJ, et al. UK malaria treatment guidelines. J Infect 2007;54:111–21.

5. Fungladda W, Honrado ER, Thimasarn K, Kitayaporn D, Karbwang J, Kamolratanakul P, et al. Compliance with artesunate and quinine + tetracycline treatment of uncomplicated falciparum malaria in Thailand. Bull World Health Organ1998;76 Suppl 1:59–66.

6. Matok I, Gorodischer R, Koren G, Sheiner E, Wiznitzer A, Levy A. The safety of metoclopramide use in the first trimester of pregnancy. N Engl J Med2009;360:2528–35.

7. Luxemburger C, McGready R, Kham A, Morison L, Cho T, Chongsuphajaisiddhi T, et al. Effects of malaria during pregnancy on infant mortality in an area of low malaria transmission. Am J Epidemiol2001;154:459–65.

8. Looareesuwan S, Phillips RE, White NJ, Kietinun S, Karbwang J, Rackow C, et al. Quinine and severe falciparum malaria in late pregnancy. Lancet1985;2:4–8.

9. McGready R, Cho T, Hkirijaroen L, Simpson J, Chongsuphajaisiddhi T, White NJ, et al. Quinine and mefloquine in the treatment of multidrug-resistant *Plasmodium falciparum* malaria in pregnancy. Ann Trop Med Parasitol1998;92:643–53.

10. McGready R, Keo NK, Villegas L, White NJ, Looareesuwan S, Nosten F. Artesunate-atovaquone-proguanil rescue treatment of multidrug-resistant *Plasmodium falciparum* malaria in pregnancy: a preliminary report. Trans R Soc Trop Med Hyg 2003;97:592–4.

11. Rijken MJ, McGready R, Boel ME, Barends M, Proux S, Pimanpanarak M, et al. Dihydro-artemisinin-piperaquine rescue treatment of multidrug-resistant *Plasmodium falciparum* malaria in pregnancy: a preliminary report. Am J Trop Med Hyg 2008;78:543–5.

12. Adam I, Ali DM, Elbashir MI. Manifestations of falciparum malaria in pregnant women of Eastern Sudan. Saudi Med J 2004;25:1947–50.

13. Krishnan A, Karnad DR. Severe falciparum malaria: an important cause of multiple organ failure in Indian intensive care unit patients. Crit Care Med 2003;31:2278–84.

14. Dorman EK, Shulman CE, Kingdom J, Bulmer JN, Mwendwa J, Peshu N, et al. Impaired uteroplacental blood flow in pregnancies complicated by falciparum malaria. Ultrasound Obstet Gynecol 2002;19:165–70.

15. CE. Shulman et al. Malaria in pregnancy: adverse effects on hemoglobin levels and birthweight in primigravidae and multigravidae. Tropical Medicine and International Health volume 6 no 10 pp 770±778 October 2001.

16. Piper C, Brabin BJ, Alpers MP. Higher risk of postpartum hemorrhage in malarious than in non-malarious areas of Papua New Guinea. Int J Gynecol Obstet2001;72:77–78.

17. Ernest A. Tako, Ainong Zhou, Julienne Lohoue, Robert Leke, Diane Wallace Taylor, Androse F. G. Leke. Risk Factors For Placental Malaria And Its Effect On Pregnancy Outcome In Yaounde, Cameroon. Am. J. Trop. Med. Hyg., 72(3), 2005, pp. 236–242.

18. McGready R, Davison BB, Stepniewska K, Cho T, Shee H, Brockman A, et al. The Effects of *Plasmodium falciparum* and *P. vivax* infections on placental histopathology in an area of low malaria transmission. Am J Trop Med Hyg 2004;70:398–407.

19

Dengue in Pregnancy

Namrata Mehta, Reena Wani, Shruti Thar

Dengue is an arboviral infection with high morbidity and mortality. The word "Dengue" in Swahili means "bone breaking fever" or the word for "walk of Dandie" in Spanish.[1] The disease was so named by Benjamin Rush in 1779. Presently about 40% of the world's population is at risk. About 50–100 million cases occur every year of which 500,000 require admission and 2.5% die.[1] Dengue fever has become an endemic in major cities of our country. In conditions with compromised immunity like pregnancy the consequences are known to be devastating for all.

ETIOLOGY

Dengue is caused by antigenically distinct serotypes belonging to genus flavivirus, single stranded RNA virus, DEN-1,2,3 and 4.[2] The vector for all the subtypes is primarily female mosquito Aedes aegypti and Aedes albopictus. This breed is known to be found in fresh water pools or artificial collections near human habitats. The mosquito is known to be a daytime feeder. The virion is known to consist of 3 structural proteins plus a lipoprotein envelope and 7 non-structural proteins of which NS1 is of diagnostic and pathological significance. Infection with anyone serotype gives lifelong immunity to that particular serotype, however, cross protection to other serotypes lasts only a few months. Some studies have shown that either the DEN-1 or DEN-2 serotype may result in more severe infection.

PATHOPHYSIOLOGY[2,3]

The virus enters human body through mosquito bite, spreads to all organs and multiplies. It is then released from these organs and infects white blood cells. There is a massive release of pyrogens and chemokines which results in symptoms of dengue.

Primary infection is usually benign in nature, however, secondary infection with a different serotype or multiple infections with different serotypes may cause severe infection that can be classified as Dengue hemorrhagic fever or Dengue shock syndrome depending on the clinical signs.

Proliferation of memory T cells and production of pro-inflammatory T cells leads to vascular endothelial cell dysfunction which results in plasma leakage. This is the hallmark of dengue hemorrhagic fever (DHF) and dengue shock syndrome (DSS). Thus there is a rise in hematocrit, hypoalbuminemia and development of pleural effusion or ascites. In severe infection, there is a loss of intravascular fluid leading to tissue hypoperfusion resulting in lactic acidosis, hypoglycemia, hypocalcemia and finally multiple organ failure.

Infants can develop severe dengue infection during a primary infection (which is usually benign in nature) due to transplacental transfer of maternal antibodies from an immune mother which subsequently amplifies the infant immune response to primary infection.

WHO CLASSIFICATION[2]

Symptomatic

- Undifferentiated fever (viral syndrome)
- Dengue fever
  - With hemorrhagic fever (unusual manifestations)
  - Without hemorrhage
- Dengue hemorrhagic fever with plasma leakage
  - Without shock
  - Dengue shock syndrome
- Expanded dengue syndrome/isolated organopathy (unusual manifestation)
- Asymptomatic

Incubation period: 2–7 days

CLINICAL FEATURES[2,3]

Dengue virus infection is known to cause a range of severe and non-severe infection.

1. Fever of recent onset is hallmark of the disease. It is usually abrupt in onset with very high spikes persisting for 4 or more days.
2. Diffuse skin flushing or rash on face, neck and chest usually appear on 3rd or 4th day. This rash may blanch when pressed and gradually resolves.
3. Headache (usually frontal), retro-orbital pain, severe backache, myalgia and arthralgia.
4. Gastrointestinal symptoms such as anorexia, nausea and vomiting, abdominal pain and loss of taste are common symptoms.
5. Hemorrhagic signs which are uncommon such as petechiae, purpura, epistaxis, gingival bleeding, malaena, hematemesis, vaginal bleeding or bleeding from venepucture.
6. Lethargy or restlessness

7. Hepatomegaly
8. Abdominal distension
9. Pleuritic chest pain, cough, dyspnea
10. Signs of circulatory collapse–cold and clammy hands, rapid and weak pulse, reduced urine output

Pregnancy does not affect the severity of dengue. It depends on previous sensitization. However, dengue may be confused with HELLP syndrome or gestational thrombocytopenia.

Effect of dengue on pregnancy includes severe bleeding (antepartum, intrapartum and postpartum), abortion, low birth weight babies, preterm deliveries and maternal death. There was a systematic review[4] of published studies to assess effect of dengue and pregnancy outcomes which showed that there is a risk of preterm birth, low birth weight, pre-eclampsia and cesarean section. The risk of vertical transmission was between 15 and 64% as suggested in that study.

INVESTIGATIONS[2,5]

1. Full blood count–leucopenia with neutropenia occurs as early as 2nd day of fever and persists till febrile period. Thrombocytopenia is typical of dengue fever. Hematocrit rises by about 10% due to dehydration.
2. Liver function tests—elevated liver enzymes AST and ALT.
3. Hypoalbuminemia <3.5 g/dl support diagnosis of DHF/DSS.
4. RT-PCR can be ordered within first 5 days of infection. Results are available in 8–12 hours depending on laboratory availability of tests. Disadvantage is that it is expensive, requires laboratory facilities and cannot distinguish between primary and secondary infection.
5. NS1 antigen detection through ELISA is useful in early diagnosis and can be ordered between day 1–9 of infection. Disadvantage is not as sensitive as RT-PCR.

6. IgM and IgG antibody can be detected by ELISA test after first 5 days of fever. IgM:IgG ratio of <1:2 suggests secondary infection.
7. Coagulation studies—may be useful in management of DHF/DSS.
8. Chest X-ray—in case of suspected pleural effusion
9. Abdominal ultrasound—in case of suspected ascites.

WHO diagnostic: Suggested dengue case classification and levels of severity[2]
Probable dengue/presumptive diagnosis
- Live in or travel to dengue endemic areas
- Fever and 2 of the following:
  - Nausea/vomiting and anorexia
  - Rash
  - Aches and pains
  - Warning signs
  - Leucopenia
  - Positive tourniquet test
- Laboratory confirmed dengue

Warning signs requiring strict observation and medical intervention include:
- Abdominal pain or tenderness
- Persistent vomiting
- Clinical fluid accumulation
- Mucosal bleed
- Lethargy/restlessness
- Liver enlargement >2 cm
- Laboratory—increase in hematocrit with decrease in platelet count

Severe dengue is defined as patients with any of the following features:
- Severe plasma leakage with shock and/or fluid accumulation with respiratory distress
- Severe hemorrhage
- Severe organ impairment

WHO: LABORATORY CRITERIA FOR DIAGNOSIS OF DHF/DSS

- Rapidly developing severe thrombocytopenia <100,000 cells/mm^3

- Decreased WBC and neutrophils
- Elevated hematocrit (>20% rise)
- Hypoalbuminemia
- Elevated LFT's

GRADING OF SEVERITY OF DENGUE HEMORRHAGIC FEVER

Grade	Symptoms and signs	Laboratory
I	Fever and hemorrhagic manifestation (positive tourniquet test) and evidence of plasma leakage	Thrombocytopenia <100,000 cmm, hematocrit rise ≥ 20%
II	Grade I plus spontaneous bleeding	Thrombocytopenia <100,000 cmm, hematocrit rise ≥ 20%
III	Grade I or II plus circulatory failure	Thrombocytopenia <100,000 cmm, hematocrit rise ≥ 20%
IV	Grade III plus profound shock	Thrombocytopenia <100,000 cmm, hematocrit rise ≥ 20%

DIFFERENTIAL DIAGNOSIS

1. Chikungunya fever
2. Malaria
3. Leptospirosis
4. Meningococcal infection
5. Typhoid
6. Rickettsial infection

TREATMENT[2]

There is no specific treatment for dengue, but appropriate medical care frequently saves the lives of patients with more severe dengue hemorrhagic fever. The most effective way to combat viral transmission is to combat the disease carrying mosquitoes.

There is a need to triage patients. Ones with any sign suggestive of severe infection need admission and observation. Some patients can be treated on OPD basis. However, one should do well to bore that dengue in pregnancy can get severe and critical and it is worth admitting these patients for observation and monitoring. Home management will include tepid sponging with paracetamol, adequate hydration and bed rest. Daily or alternate day follow up with CBC is done depending on clinical assessment.

A stepwise approach to the management of dengue (based on WHO guidelines)

Step I. Overall assessment

I.1 History, including information on symptoms, past medical and family history

I.2 Physical examination, including full physical and mental assessment

I.3 Investigation, including routine laboratory and dengue-specific laboratory

Step II. Diagnosis, assessment of disease phase and severity

Step III. Management

III.1 Disease notification

III.2 Management decisions. Depending on the clinical manifestations and other circumstances, patients may:

- Be sent home (Group A)
- Be referred for in-hospital management (Group B)
- Require emergency treatment and urgent referral (Group C).

Warning signs for admission (Group B)

- Persisting or worsening of symptoms
- Vomiting and not tolerating orals
- Severe abdominal pain
- Lethargy and or restlessness
- Bleeding
- Giddiness
- Pale, cold and clammy hands
- Less or no urine output

Management of DHF (Group C) includes:

1. Frequent monitoring of symptoms and signs.
2. Adequate perfusion with IVF fluids to maintain input and output.

3. Monitoring of temperature, pulse, blood pressure, respiratory rate and saturation.
4. Serial blood tests for monitoring.
5. Correction abnormal laboratory results.

There is a retrospective study[6] conducted in a tertiary center in Coimbatore where the author suggests that the most frequent complication with dengue in pregnancy is thrombocytopenia which can be severe enough to require platelet transfusion. They have noted that dengue in pregnancy is managed conservatively as in non-pregnant state and no associated poor neonatal outcome except low birth weight.

There was a another case series study done in Sri Lanka[7] wherein the authors concluded that Dengue in pregnancy requires early diagnosis and treatment. One needs to be alert of the possibility of dengue in pregnancy so as to undertake appropriate monitoring and management. However, appropriate studies regarding effects and management of dengue in pregnancy is still lacking.

Prevention

Regions with endemic dengue virus infection should have preventive measures in place to prevent spread of infection. Various methods include:

1. Regularly removing all sources of stagnant water to prevent breeding of mosquitos.
2. Preventing mosquito bites by covering exposed areas of skin, mosquito repellants, coils and nets.

A tetravalent vaccine is currently being developed and may be available in the future.

REFERENCES

1. http://www.searo.who.int/publications/journals/seajph/seajphv3n1p22.pdf
2. World Health Organisation, Regional Office for South-East Asia. Comprehensive guidelines for prevention and control of dengue and dengue hemorrhagic fever—revised and expanded edition 2011. http:??www.searo.who.int/
3. http://www.cdc.gov/dengue/symptoms/

4. "Maternal Dengue and pregnancy outcomes: a systematic review" Pouliot SH, Xiong X , Obstet Gynecol Surv 2010 Feb;65(2):107–18

5. Laayanarooj S, Vaughn DW, Nimmannitya A, et al. Early clinical and laboratory indicators of acute dengue illness. J.Infect. Dis.1997;176:313–321.

6. TV Chitra, Seetha Panicker Maternal and fetal outcome of Dengue fever in pregnancy, J. Vector borne disease 48, Dec 2011, pp210–213 http://www.mrcindia.org/journal/issues/484210.pdf

7. Sampath Kariyawasam, Hemantha Senanayake Dengue infections in pregnancy : Case series from a tertiary care hospital in Sri Lanka J Infect Dev Ctries 2010;4(11):767–775 *www.jidc.org › Home › Vol 4, No 11 › Kariyawasam*

20

Swine Flu in Pregnancy

Shreya Prabhoo, Reena Wani

INTRODUCTION

Swine Flu as it is very commonly known is an infection with a virus named Influenza A H1N1. It is a novel strain of the Influenza A virus. The outbreak of Swine Flu occurred first in Mexico in the year 2009 after which there were growing number of cases throughout the globe and was declared as a global pandemic by the WHO. This virus has now emerged predominantly and affects patients every influenza season.

This virus is an Orthomyxovirus. It is an enveloped virus with the characteristic spike-like viral glycoproteins called Haemagglutinin and Neuraminidase, hence their description H1N1. It has tremendous ability to mutate. It contains a mixture of genetic material from human, pig and bird flu virus. It is a new variety of flu to which humans have not had much immunity.

The influenza virus is known for its ability to mutate. This new strain appears to be a result of reassortment of human influenza and swine influenza viruses, in all four different strains of subtype H1N1.

This influenza typically affects the age group between 5 and 65 years.[1]

The virus is highly contagious and is contracted by aerosol transmission by inhaling the droplets from an infected person coughing and sneezing or by touching one's mouth and nose after contact with a contaminated surface.

SYMPTOMS OF SWINE FLU

- Highly contagious during the first 5 days of illness
- High fever usually above 38°C
- Cough, sore throat
- Headaches, aching muscles
- Chills and fever
- Exhaustion on fatigue
- Diarrhea or a stomach upset
- The median duration of symptoms is 7 days.
- Usually patients who are affected suffer a mild viral illness, and make a full recovery.

Patients suffering from the following symptoms are more likely to be admitted to the intensive care unit. These are:

- Dyspnea, respiratory rate >30 per minute
- Requirement for supplemental oxygen, respiratory support
- Pneumonia on admission
- Tachycardia
- Altered conscious level

RISK GROUPS

- Age <5 years, socially deprived, underlying medical problems
- 16–64 years age group with associated co-morbidities (cardiac disease, renal disease)
- Diabetes
- Immunosuppression from cytotoxic drugs or autoimmune disease, Asthma, HIV infection
- Morbid obesity
- Pregnancy

EFFECTS OF PREGNANCY

Pregnancy induces a unique challenge for the maternal immune system, as it has to tolerate the semiallogenic fetus and maintain a strong immune response against invading pathogens. Influenza viruses take advantage of these alterations in maternal immune system thus putting them at a higher risk of developing pulmonary complications, especially in the second and third trimester. There is no evidence to suggest that pregnant women are more susceptible to the flu virus.[2] The enlarging uterus presses on the diaphragm and together with changes in the lungs such as reduced tidal volume, congestion and localized edema, make the woman more prone to complications such as pneumonia and Adult Respiratory Distress Syndrome (ARDS). Recent reports have shown that the percentage of pregnant patients requiring transfer to ICU within each trimester is similar (27, 25, 24%); and the death rate amongst patients within each gestational age group is also uniform (10, 6, 9%). This may imply that outcome in severely ill pregnant women is independent of gestational age after severe illness is established.[3]

INDICATIONS FOR HOSPITALIZATION

Pregnant women with swine flu are four times more likely to be hospitalized: There is 3 × increase risk of preterm delivery, 5 × increases in stillbirth rate and increased risk of maternal death. Younger pregnant women and women with co-morbidities are at higher risk of complications. If there is a delay in start of antiviral treatment, hospitalization is required.

GENERAL TREATMENT[4, 5]

There are 2 types of antiviral drugs known to be effective in swine flu:
1. Oseltamivir (Tamiflu)—administered orally.
2. Zanamivir (Relenza)—available as inhaler (Diskhaler).

They are neuraminidase inhibitors and act by preventing the virus from budding and escaping from the host cells. It acts directly on the respiratory tract with no absorption in the blood stream, thus being the drug of choice in pregnant women. If patient cannot tolerate inhaler as in cases of severe asthma or pneumonia, then oral Tamiflu can be given. If patient presents with flu-like symptoms, i.e. cold, fever, sore throat, then azithromycin is started. Throat swab is sent for A H1N1 testing. If the throat swab is positive patients are started on oseltamivir for 5 days. If patient has dyspnea, pneumonia in the first visit, then patient is admitted and started with oseltamivir immediately. Pregnant women with flu-like symptoms are admitted and started on zanamivir or oseltamivir directly. Throat swab is sent for diagnoses though. Pregnant women admitted should be managed jointly by the obstetrician and physician deciding the place of management with a clear plan set out from the outset. Women who require respiratory support may be managed in the ICU with close monitoring by obstetricians. If the women goes in labor and intensive care facilities are available in the labor room, then she should be shifted to the delivery unit or patient should be managed in the ICU itself.

STANDARD DOSAGES

Oseltamivir: For adolescents (13 to 17 years of age) and adults the recommended oral dose (based on data from studies in typical uncomplicated influenza) is 75 mg oseltamivir twice daily for 5 days. *Zanamivir* is indicated for treatment of influenza in adults and children (> 5 years). The recommended dose for treatment of adults and children from the age of 5 years (based on data from studies in typical uncomplicated influenza) is two inhalations (i.e. 2 × 5 mg) twice daily for 5 days.

ANTENATAL CORTICOSTEROIDS

Current obstetric practice is to administer corticosteroids, e.g. 2 doses of betamethasone

12 mg, 24 hours apart or 4 doses of Dexamethasone 6 mg, 6 hours apart to promote fetal lung maturity in cases of threatened pre-term labor or where a decision of premature delivery of fetus is to be made for maternal or fetal reasons. The effects on the maternal immune system from a single course of corticosteroids are unclear but the evidence does not suggest that it results in sufficient immuno-suppression to cause maternal harm or exacerbation of infection.[6] The administration of corticosteroids is important for the promotion of fetal lung maturity, and the benefits outweigh the risks. Although high dose of steroids for treatment of pulmonary complications is not recommended as it may lead to immuno-suppression and prolonged viral shedding.

DELIVERY

Most pregnant women with symptoms of influenza will be able to tolerate labor with adequate pain relief and hydration. In most of the cases, the decision to deliver will be made for an obstetric indication. In the case of a critically ill woman close to term, woman can be delivered by cesarean section to help mechanical ventilation of the lungs to improve recovery. This should be done once her clinical condition is stabilized and other potential complications such as coagulopathy have been excluded or corrected. The decision is made in conjunction with the obstetric, critical care and neonatal teams. In case of a patient whose elective cesarean section was planned before, should be started on anti-viral and allowed to settle at least for 5 days until completion of treatment. This will allow her to recover and reduce the chances of respiratory complications.

POSTNATAL PERIOD

Women in the postnatal period are at lower risk of respiratory complications as the effect of the gravid uterus pressing on the diaphragm has been removed. However, complications due to secondary infection may still occur and there is a risk of transmission to the newborn infant. Mothers should observe strict hygiene and should be offered anti-viral treatment, oseltamivir is a safe drug during breastfeeding. Breastfeeding should be encouraged and continued as long as possible as (i) it gives the appropriate nutrition for health and promotes mother–child bonding, (ii) antibody rich colostrum helps in the immunity of the neonate. If mother cannot breastfeed directly, breast milk should be expressed and fed to the neonate.

PROPHYLAXIS

The best way of reducing the risk of transmission of the virus is to observe good respiratory hygiene, i.e. covering the mouth and nose while coughing or sneezing. Wash hands frequently with soap and water. An infected person should avoid going to crowded places. Pre- or post-exposure prophylaxis with antivirals has been shown to be effective in preventing the infection but at the same time it may inhibit the development of immunity and prolonged, repeated prophylaxis may result in development of resistance. Prophylaxis is recommended for very high risk individuals including pregnant women in whom risk of development of severe disease with complications is higher.[6]

Public Guidelines by Indian Medical Association[7]

- Prevention is the key by: Avoid touching face (mouth and nose) with your hands
- Avoid touching or having close proximity with any person who is coughing or has cold/sneezing
- Avoid shaking hands and patients who have symptoms should stay indoors
- Avoid going to office/schools or in crowded locations till the time their symptoms subside.
- Most swine flu patients can be managed at home based on the symptoms.
- Drugs (Chemoprophylaxis) are only recommended for symptomatic individuals (on the discretion of a doctor) and pregnant

ladies or those suffering from concomitant illnesses (like diabetes, cardiac or respiratory illnesses or end-organ failures).

VACCINES

The vaccine contains inactivated H1N1 virus that has been developed from the bird flu H5N1. Most people do not have immunity to this virus. This inactivated virus does not cause any harm to the mother or fetus, but at the same time it develops active immunity. The antibody response to vaccines in pregnant women has been shown to be as effective as in non-pregnant women.[8] Influenza vaccines can prevent flu caused by human strains, which is recommended by IMA Guidelines 2015 for:

- Children above 6 months
- Adults > 50 years of age
- Patients with pulmonary, cardiovascular, renal, hepatic, neurologic, hematologic disorders and diabetes mellitus
- Pregnant females and healthcare providers. The inactivated vaccine can be given to the above groups. The Live attenuated influenza vaccine (intranasal spray) can be given only to persons aged 2–49 years (not to pregnant females).[7]

Influenza Foundation of India (IFI)[9] aims to promote awareness of influenza among healthcare professionals, with the intention of enhancing control measures and boosting pandemic preparedness in the India region. Influenza is a public health problem of collective concern to the community and IFI has defined objectives:

i. To improve knowledge on influenza disease and its epidemiology in India
ii. To disseminate unbiased scientific information on influenza to the medical community and the public
iii. To promote influenza pandemic preparedness activity in India
iv. To co-ordinate news and activities related to influenza, between the private sector and government
v. To produce educational and scientific material for the medical community and the public. To achieve these objectives, IFI has prepared a detailed white paper on influenza.

CONCLUSION

The influenza A H1N1 virus has emerged as a predominant virus in the seasonal influenza season. The population at high risk being younger population, pregnant and immuno-compromised individuals. Mostly patients make a full recovery after a mild flu. However, pregnant women need to be actively treated from the start as they are likely to develop complications. Strict hygiene should be maintained to prevent the spread of the virus. Early medical advice and treatment can prevent morbidity and mortality because of swine flu.

REFERENCES

1. Jamieson DJ, Honein MA, Rasmussen SA, et al. H1N1 2009 influenza virus infection during pregnancy in the USA. Lancet. 2009;374:451–458. doi: 10.1016/S0140-6736(09)61304-0.
2. Stirrat GM. Pregnancy and immunity. BMJ. 1994;308:1385–1386.
3. Siston AM, Rasmussen SA, Honein MA, et al. Pandemic 2009 influenza A (H1N1) virus illness among pregnant women in the United States. JAMA 2010;303(15)1517–25.
4. Clinical management of human infection with pandemic (H1N1) 2009: revised guidance. World Health Organization, November 2009. Available at: http://www.who.int/csr/resources/publications/swineflu/clinical_management/en/index.html.
5. Pharmacological Management of Pandemic Influenza A (H1N1). World Health Organization 2009 Part I: Recommendations. Rev Feb 2010.
6. Boon H. Lim, Tahir A. Mahmood. Influenza A H1N1 2009 (Swine Flu) and Pregnancy. J Obstet Gynaecol India. 2011 Aug; 61(4):386–393.
7. Indian Medical Association. "Treat Swine Flu like Ordinary Flu". Prakash et al. Public Guidelines, 1st January 2015.
8. Meeting of the Strategic Advisory Group of Experts on immunization, April 2010—conclusions and recommendations. Weekly Epidemiological Report, World Health Organization. 2010:85; 197–212.
9. http://www.influenzafoundationofindia.org/

21

Herpes in Pregnancy

Chitra Nayak

The term "herpes" in pregnancy includes infections caused by human herpes viruses 1, 2 and 3 (varicella zoster virus causing herpes zoster) in pregnant women as well as "herpes gestationis" (pemphigoid gestationis) which is an immunologically mediated pregnancy specific dermatosis and not caused by herpesviruses.

Human herpes viruses (HHV) are known to be eight in number, of these HHV 1, 2 and 3 cause conditions named herpes—herpes simplex viruses 1 and 2 correspond to HHV1 and HHV2 while the varicella-zoster virus which causes chickenpox as the primary infection and herpes zoster on reactivation is HHV3.

HERPES SIMPLEX

The herpes simplex viruses (HSV) 1 and 2 are ubiquitous, usually causing orolabial and genital herpes. Genital herpes is perhaps the most common sexually transmitted infection worldwide. The primary infection of Herpes simplex virus is one where there are no pre-existing antibodies to HSV1 or HSV2. A non-primary initial infection means infection with one HSV type in an individual who already has antibodies to the other HSV type—there may or may not be symptoms of either or both. Latency of the virus in sensory ganglia is common to both HSV1 and HSV2. Reactivation of latent virus leads to recurrent manifestations of infection or asymptomatic shedding.

Genital infections are usually caused by HSV2, but in the US, Canada and the UK, HSV1 now accounts for the majority of genital herpes infections. Viral transmission occurs even during asymptomatic shedding. Direct contact with contaminated saliva or other secretions is the main cause of spread of HSV1 while sexual contact is main cause for HSV2 spread. Virus replicates at mucocutaneous site of infection, travels to dorsal root ganglia by retrograde axonal flow and remains latent until reactivation. Reactivation occurs either spontaneously or by a trigger such as emotional stress, ultraviolet light, fever, local tissue damage or immunosuppression due to any cause.[1]

Clinical Features[1]

The primary infection becomes symptomatic 3 to 7 days after exposure with tender lymphadenopathy, malaise, anorexia and fever being the prodrome before mucocutaneous lesions which could be heralded by localized pain, tenderness, burning or tingling. Cutaneous lesions of painful grouped usually umbilicated vesicles on an erythematous base which progress to pustules (Fig. 21.1), erosions (Fig. 21.2) or ulcers with scalloped borders. Crusting followed by resolution occurs usually within

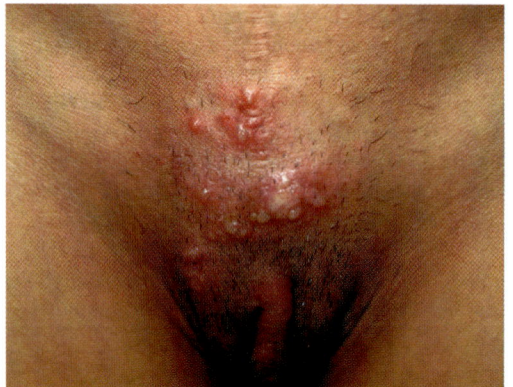

Fig. 21.1: Vesicles and vesico-pustules of genital herpes

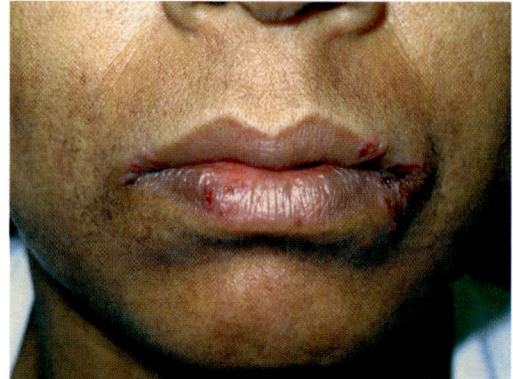

Fig. 21.3: Herpes labialis-vesicles, erosions, crusts

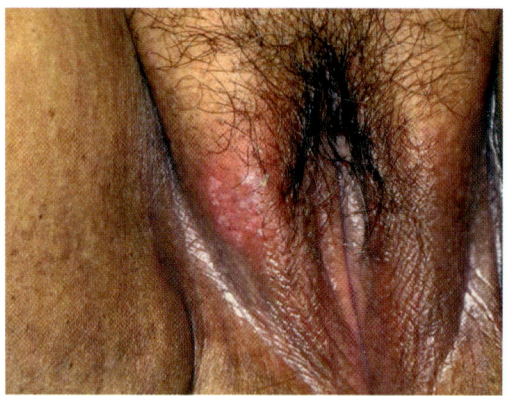

Fig. 21.2: Erosions on an erythematous base on vulva

two weeks, rarely may take as long as six weeks. Every recurrence may be preceded by a prodrome but the lesions are fewer with decreased severity and duration with recurrences.

Most primary orolabial infections are asymptomatic. Severe infections like gingivostomatitis in children and pharyngitis with a mononucleosis in adults are usually symptomatic. The commonest sites of infection are the mouth and lips (Fig. 21.3), lesions are typically seen on the buccal mucosa and gingivae. Painful oropharyngeal lesions with edema lead to drooling and dysphagia. Recurrent lesions are seen usually on the vermilion border of the lip while the perioral skin, nasal mucosa, oral mucosa over hard palate and cheek are less common sites.

Primary and non-primary genital herpes infections may present with excruciatingly painful erosive vulvitis or vaginitis. Lesions may involve the cervix, buttocks and perineum causing inguinal adenopathy and dysuria with systemic complaints and complications. Extragenital lesions occur in about a fifth of the patients and urinary retention and aseptic meningitis in more than a tenth of affected women. The lesional involvement, regional lymphadenopathy and fever are milder in recurrent disease. A few vesicles may appear on the buttocks or genitalia which resolve within a week. Subclinical viral shedding is also known to occur. The frequency of recurrences decreases over the years.

In patients with atopic dermatitis or pre-existing dermatoses like pemphigus, burns, mycosis fungoides, or Darier's disease the herpes simplex virus can cause eczema herpeticum or Kaposi's varicelliform eruption due to the rapid dissemination of the virus in areas of disrupted skin barrier. There is fever, malaise and lymphadenopathy with mono-morphic, discrete, punched out erosions with hemorrhagic crusts, intact vesicles are less common. Bacterial superinfection or dissemi-nated herpes infection may further complicate the picture.

Herpetic whitlow presents with pain, swelling and vesicular lesions which recur at same location, mainly in children due to digital-genital contact. Dental and medical personnel who previously did not use gloves could develop it and it was often misdiagnosed as paronychia.

Herpes simplex folliculitis is usually caused by HSV1 and is seen as follicular vesicles and pustules in immunocompromised individuals. Severe and chronic HSV infections present as chronic, enlarging ulcerations affecting multiple sites and may coalesce. Verrucous, exophytic or pustular lesions may also occur. Mucosal involvement of the oral cavity which may also involve the whole gastrointestinal tract may also occur.

Ocular HSV infection can result in keratoconjuctivitis with eyelid edema, photophobia, tearing, chemosis and preauricular lymphadenopathy. Branching dendritic lesions of cornea can lead to ulceration and corneal scarring, rupture of globe and blindness. Herpes encephalitis presents with fever, altered mental status, bizarre behavior and localized neurologic findings.

If a pregnant woman has primary HSV2 infection or disseminated infection, she is more likely to transmit HSV to the neonate than if she has recurrent infection. Mothers of infants born with HSV rarely have overt HSV infection at delivery. Transplacental or ascending infection by HSV due to prolonged rupture of membranes is rare. Infection may be transmitted post-natally to the neonate by contact with lesions of herpes on genital and non-genital sites of the mother or other individuals.[2] A mother who has had primary genital HSV infection during pregnancy is more likely to have asymptomatic viral shedding at delivery[3] than one who has had recurrent HSV infection.[4] To prevent neonatal herpes, cesarean section must be done within four hours of rupture of membranes.[5] Non-genital primary infection with HSV1 in the mother during pregnancy may or may not have serious adverse effects on the fetus.[6,7]

Neonatal Herpes[1]

The incidence of neonatal herpes varies from one case per 12500 to 1 per 1700 live births. (Corey L, Wald A Maternal and neonatal herpes simplex virus infections. New Engl J Med 361(14): 1376–1385, 2009). It is estimated to be about 1:50,000 births in the UK. (bolognia). The neonate falls in a special category of the immunodeficient host. The risk of neonatal herpes is defined by the category of maternal infection. A 25–50% risk of neonatal infection in vaginally delivered babies exists in mothers with primary genital infection. Up to 50–80% of neonatal HSV infections occur due to this. This risk of transmission is less than 3% when there is recurrent maternal infection as transplacental antibodies may decrease risk of transmission.

Factors which increase risk of neonatal herpes are vaginal delivery, presence of cervical HSV infection, use of invasive monitors, prolonged rupture of membranes and if HSV is isolated from genital tract. Manifestations of neonatal herpes are as skin, eye and oral involvement, encephalitis and disseminated disease. In case of limited mucocutaneous involvement, there could be vesiculation or subtle blistering and peeling of skin with inflamed and ulcerated mucosae. Encephalitis and disseminated disease account for more than 50% cases of neonatal herpes. Lethargy, seizures, respiratory distress, hepato-splenomegaly with hepatitis and thromocytopenia are features of disseminated disease. More than a fifth of neonates with neurologic and disseminated disease do not develop cutaneous vesicles. In untreated neonatal herpes, the mortality is 65%, 6% is mortality even in treated babies with encephalitis and about 90% of neonatal herpes with CNS infection will have neurologic deficits. Most babies with skin, eye and oral disease survive if treated and are seen to be developing normally at one year. The babies with disseminated disease have 30% mortality even if treated and about

80% of survivors are seen to develop normally at one year.

Diagnosis[1]

Viral culture, direct fluorescent antibody assays, molecular techniques and serology can be used to diagnose HSV infections. The Tzanck smear (a cytologic smear from the floor or edges of a freshly unroofed vesicle) shows the viral cytopathic effect on epithelial cells of multinucleate giant cells, which however are seen in herpes simplex infections, herpes zoster and varicella. Tzanck smear and biopsy do not differentiate HSV1 from HSV2. Direct fluorescence antibody test has greater sensitivity and can also distinguish between herpes simplex and varicella zoster viruses, the added advantage is a rapid turnaround time. Viral culture gives results in 2–5 days. Polymerase chain reaction is a rapid, sensitive and specific method to detect HSV DNA from skin and other organs especially cerebrospinal fluid.

The Western blot which is 99% sensitive and specific is the gold standard for serologic tests for HSV antibodies. It is useful to confirm primary infections but recurrent infection may not show significant changes in titre.

Treatment[1]

Aciclovir is proven effective in primary herpes simplex infections in the dose 200 mg five times daily for 5–7 days, 400 mg thrice daily is given for recurrences. Antiviral treatment of herpes during pregnancy can reduce the risk of preterm delivery versus not treating with antivirals.[8] Topical acyclovir cream is not useful. In case of severe or disseminated infection in adults, neonatal herpes is treated with high doses of intravenous acyclovir, viz. 20mg/kg/day in three divided doses for 2–3 weeks. Valaciclovir 500 mg twice daily for 3 days, or famciclovir 250 mg twice daily for 5 days may also be used. Foscarnet or cidofovir may be used in suspected acyclovir resistance.

VARICELLA AND HERPES ZOSTER

The varicella-zoster virus causes chickenpox as a primary infection and herpes zoster as the late reactivation of the infection. The primary infection is predominantly acquired in childhood and 95% adults have antibodies to the virus. Direct contact and respiratory transmission cause the primary infection after 10–21 days incubation period. Individuals are infectious from just before onset of the rash until the last lesion has crusted over.

Clinical features: Clinically, flu-like symptoms followed by a rash that is centripetal and goes through the stages of erythematous papules turning into papulovesicles which then evolve into vesicles before crusting over. Adults have a severe infection (Fig. 21.4) and half the mortality of varicella happens in non-immune adults, mainly due to varicella pneumonia which is more severe in adults and particularly so in pregnant women. When infected, about 5% of pregnant women

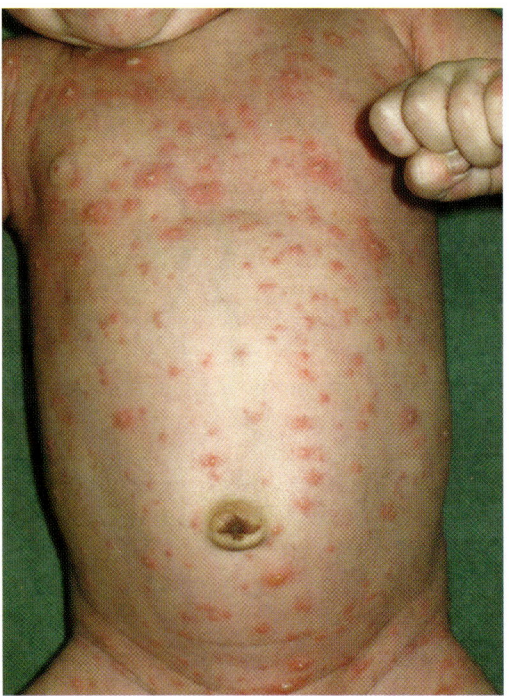

Fig. 21.4: Neonatal varicella in 21-day-old, mother had perinatal varicella

develop pneumonitis, which becomes symptomatic about 3–5 days into the illness. There is fever, tachypnea, dry cough, dyspnea and pleuritic pain with nodular infiltrates seen in the lungs on radiography. Though the pneumonia resolves along with the skin lesions, fever and compromise of lung function may persist for weeks.

Reactivation of varicella infection causes herpes zoster (also called shingles). Herpes zoster is less contagious than chickenpox, the affected patient is contagious from the time of the appearance of the first blister until all blisters are crusted. There is not much evidence to show that herpes zoster causes congenital malformations.

Pain, either sharply localized or diffuse, is usually the first manifestation of herpes zoster, preceding the eruption by 1–3 days. It is accompanied by fever, headache, malaise and tenderness on areas of skin corresponding to one or more dorsal roots. Grouped red papules which soon turn vesicular develop along one or more contiguous dermatomes, involving the mucous membranes with the dermatome also. The vesicles may turn pustular or crust over directly. Draining lymph nodes are enlarged and tender.

If a woman has chickenpox in the first half of pregnancy, the fetus may develop congenital varicella syndrome which includes chorioretinitis, microphthalmia, cerebral cortical atrophy, growth retardation, hydronephrosis and skin or bone defects.[10] A study by Enders et al[11] revealed that when maternal infection occurred before 13 weeks of gestation, only 0.4% neonates had congenital varicella while between 13 and 20 weeks 2% neonates were affected. No evidence of congenital infection was found after 20 weeks gestation. No serological evidence of intrauterine infection was found in infants whose mothers had herpes zoster in pregnancy. No cases of congenital varicella syndrome or zoster in infancy occurred in 97 pregnant women who had varicella after

post-exposure prophylaxis with anti-varicella zoster immunoglobulin.

Management

The diagnosis of varicella and herpeszoster is clinical. A Tzanck smear from the floor of a ruptured vesicle will reveal the viral cytopathic effect of multinucleate giant cells, tissue culture may grow the virus. Direct fluorescent antibody testing can be done to confirm diagnosis. Congenital varicella is diagnosed by nucleic acid amplification techniques on amniotic fluid, however, a positive result does not always lead to development of congenital infection.[12] Peripartum exposure to varicella before maternal antibodies have formed is dangerous to newborns. Between 25 to 50% get neonatal varicella (Fig. 21.5) with a 25% mortality rate. Systemic and central nervous system disease is the reason for most fatalities. To try and prevent this, varicella-zoster immune globulin is administered to neonates born to mothers with varicella 5 days before and up to 2 days after delivery.

Exposed pregnant women if not known to have had chickenpox, must be tested for varicella zoster virus serology. More than half will be positive and therefore immune. Exposed pregnant women if seronegative must be given varicella-zoster immune globulin within 96 hours of exposure in order

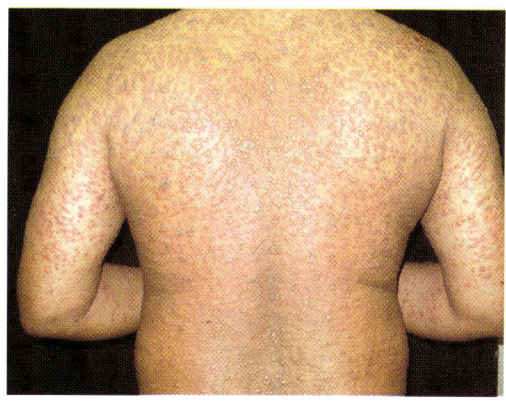

Fig. 21.5: Chickenpox in an adult-profuse vesicles

to prevent or attenuate varicella infection. If the pregnant woman develops varicella, a chest radiograph must be done to rule out pneumonitis. Intravenous acyclovir 10–15 mg/kg every eight hours is given for a week to 10 days.[13] Attenuated live virus vaccine is available and recommended to all adolescents who have not had chickenpox. Two doses are given 8 weeks apart, giving 97% seroconversion. However, vaccine induced immunity wanes with time and about 5% breakthrough infections are seen at 10 years. The vaccine should not be given to pregnant women and a woman should not become pregnant for at least two months after receiving the vaccine. However, congenital varicella syndrome or malformations have not been reported from vaccine exposed pregnancies. As the vaccine virus is not secreted in breast milk, women need not delay postpartum vaccination.

Herpes zoster is treated with acyclovir 800 mg five times daily or intravenous acyclovir 10 mg/kg per dose 8 hourly for 7–10 days. Valaciclovir 1 gm or famciclovir 500 mg thrice daily may also be used. Topical acyclovir is not useful.

HERPES GESTATIONIS (PEMPHIGOID GESTATIONIS)

Herpes gestationis is an eruption that has clinical and immunofluorescence similarities to bullous pemphigoid (BP), so pemphigoid gestationis (PG) is considered to be more appropriate nomenclature for it. Pemphigoid gestationis (herpes gestationis) is probably the least common pregnancy specific dermatosis. It is characterized by an extremely pruritic urticarial rash during late pregnancy or the immediate post-partum period which evolves into a vesiculobullous eruption. Waxing and waning of the rash during pregnancy with flare during labor and delivery is also seen.

It occurs in about 1 in 50,000 pregnancies and is associated with HLA-DR3 and HLA-DR4. A specific immunoglobulin (Ig) G against the cutaneous basement membrane zone which induces C3 (complement) deposition along the dermal-epidermal junction is the mediator of this eruption.[15]

Etiopathogenesis[14]

Cause of PG is an anti-basement membrane zone (BMZ) autoantibody that induces C3 deposition along the dermal-epidermal junction. Direct immunofluorescence infrequently finds the PG autoantibody, but complement added indirect IF reveals circulating IgG in most patients. An enzyme linked immunosorbent assay (ELISA) test is available to detect levels of this autoantibody which co-relate with disease activity. The autoantibody is an IgG1 to BP180 (typeXVII collagen). Bp180 is a 180 kDa trans-membrane protein with its N-terminal end embedded in the intracellular component of the hemi-desmosome and its C-terminal end remaining extracellular. The extracellular section consists of 15 collagenous components alternating with 16 short, non-collagenous domains. The sixteenth non-collagenous segment designated NC16A contains the BP180 immunoreactive site and is closest to the basal keratinocyte plasma membrane. It is not known what causes this autoantibody production, but as PG is seen exclusively in pregnancy, immuno-genetics is probably at play and the cross-reactivity between placental tissue and skin also plays a role. Though immunogenetic studies reveal an increase in HLA antigens DR3 and DR4 or both, patients with neither of these may have disease indistinguishable from classical PG. However, all women will have demonstrable HLA antigens. The autoantibody of PG binds to amniotic basement membrane which is derived from fetal ectoderm and antigenically similar to skin. Villous stroma of chorionic villi but not skin of women with PG show increased expression of major histocompatibility complex class II antigens (DR, DP, DQ). It is hypothesized that aberrant expression of major histocompatibility complex class II antigens (of paternal haplotype) within the placenta initiates an allogeneic response to placental BMZ which cross-reacts with skin producing pemphigoid gestationis. Pemphigoid gestationis has also been reported in association with hydatidiform moles[15] and choriocarcinomas.[16] The pemphigoid gestation is considered a paraneoplastic eruption of the choriocarcinoma. Most hydatidiform moles have diploid contribution of paternal chromosomes and contain neither amnion nor fetal tissue. There are no case reports of PG like rash in males with choriocarcinoma which consists of strictly syngeneic tissue. Placental tissue of paternal derivation is what choriocarcinoma in women is derived from, suggesting that it is not the presence of amnion but the state of partial allograph on which depends the development of pemphigoid gestationis.

Clinical Features[14]

Figure 21.6 shows that abrupt eruption of intensely pruritic urticarial lesions during late pregnancy is the usual presentation of

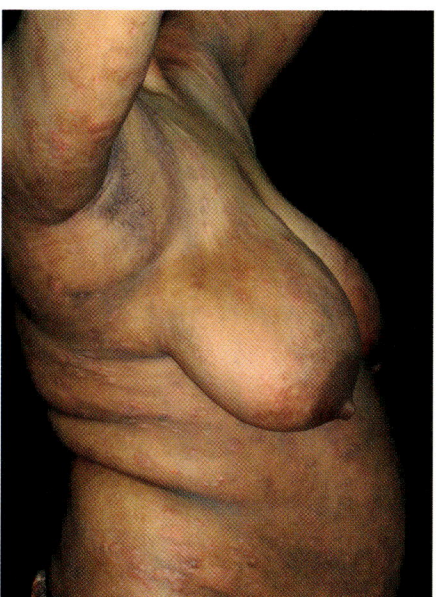

Fig. 21.6: Pemphigoid gestationis-erythematous papules, vesicles, erosions, crusts

pemphigoid gestationis. More than half the patients develop lesions first on the abdomen near the umbilicus, which progresses to a generalized pemphigoid like eruption consisting of erythematous papules, vesicles which can erode and crust, which spares only the face, mucous membranes, palms and soles. The remaining develop typical lesions on the extremities, palms and soles. About three-fourths of the patients have dramatic flares of the eruption with delivery. Often an explosive onset of the eruption during delivery may be the presenting feature in 25% of the patients.

About 10% of the neonates born to these mothers will have a mild and self-limited eruption. Even those who do not have an eruption show positive findings on immuno-fluorescence.

Differences between pemphigoid gesta-tionis and bullous pemphigoid are many. BP is a disease of the elderly with no gender bias, PG is exclusively seen in women associated with pregnancy (ortrophoblastic tissue). Association with HLA-DR3 and DR4 and a C4 null allele seen in PG is not seen in BP. Most patients of BP show positive results on indirect immunofluorescence with a high titre of anti-basement membrane zone antibody. The titre of anti-basement membrane zone antibody is so low in PG that it is detected only by adding complement or ELISA techniques. The majority to BP sera react to an intracellular 230- to 240-kDa component of the hemidesmosome while sera from most PG patients react to a 180-kDa transmembrane protein with a collagenous domain coded for on a different chromosome.

Clinically, urticarial or arcuate plaques that rapidly evolve to tense pemphigoid-lile blisters with blisters erupting on otherwise normal looking skin. It should be differentiated from pruritic urticarial papules and plaques of pregnancy which does not show the tense blisters of PG though it shows micro-vesiculation.

The first onset of pemphigoid gestationis has been reported during both primiparous and nulliparous pregnancies with and without a change in partners.

Investigations[14]

Biochemical and hematological findings are not deranged in pemphigoid gestationis. Antinuclear antibodies are absent and serum complement levels are normal. Histopathology of a vesicle classically shows a sub-epidermal vesicle with a perivascular infiltrate of lymphocytes and eosinophils (Fig. 21.7). Eosinophils may be lined up at the dermo-epidermal junctions and present abundantly within the vesicle. Many cases may show a non-specific mixed cellular infiltrate with a variable number of eosinophils.

On direct immunofluorescence(IF) of perilesional skin, finding C3 with or without Ig in a linear band along the BMZ is pathognomonic. Indirect immunofluorescence done by adding complement reveals anti-BMZ IgG in almost all patients. The PG ELISA test may replace direct IF, the antibody titres co-relate with disease severity. All patients, however, may not react with the BP180 antibody alone, if the relevant antigen is outside the NC16A site, those cases may be missed. Though thyroid dysfunction is rare,

an increased incidence of anti-thyroid antibodies has been seen in those with a history of PG.

As initial lesions of PG are urticarial, it may often be mistaken for pruritic urticarial papules and plaques of pregnancy (PUPPP). However, as vesicles and bullae develop rapidly, the diagnosis becomes evident. However, it may also be mistaken for drug eruptions or allergic contact dermatitis. Immunofluorescence or ELISA helps differentiate the various conditions and helps planning of future pregnancies. Prurigo of pregnancy and pruritic folliculitis of pregnancy are the other conditions that pemphigoid gestationis should be differentiated from.

The newborn may have lesions similar to PG but they are self-limited, not requiring any treatment. There may be an increased risk of premature or small for gestational age births, but no increase in spontaneous abortion or stillbirth has been noted. There has not been any reported increase in maternal morbidity or mortality due to pemphigoid gestationis or due to steroids used to treat it.[17] Women who have suffered from pemphigoid gestationis may suffer from secondary autoimmune disease, of which Graves' disease is most frequent.[18]

Clinical course: Pemphigoid gestationis clinical presentation and course may be very variable. Spontaneous resolution may occur as pregnancy advances but there may be a

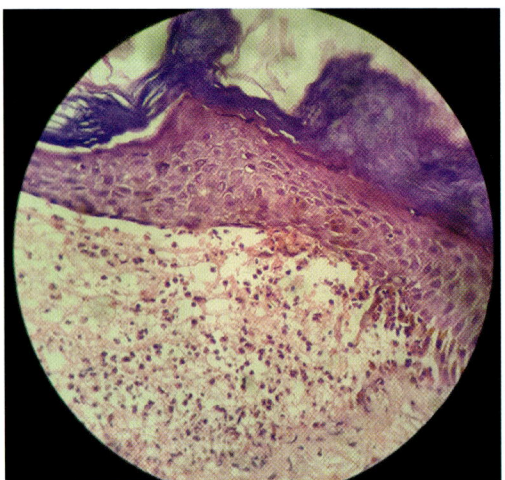

Fig. 21.7: H&E 400X, Pemphigoid gestationis—subepidermal blister with lymphocytes and plenty of eosinophils

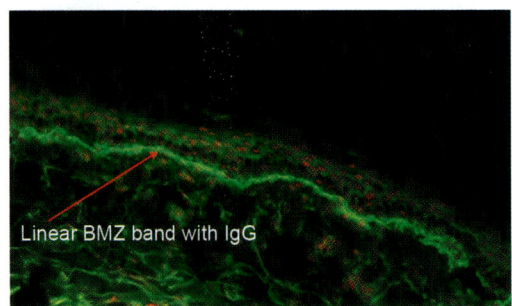

Linear BMZ band with IgG

Fig. 21.8: Direct immunofluorescence-linear deposition of IgG at dermo-epidermal junction

Algorithm for rash in pregnancy

```
                    Rash in pregnancy
                           |
            ┌──────────────┴──────────────┐
   Related to pregnancy          Unrelated coincidental
            |                       occurrence of rash
    ┌───────┴────────┐
Clinically compatible   Incompatible clinically
with pemphigoid         with pemphigoid
gestationis             gestationis
    |                        |
ELISA assay             Other skin eruptions
    |                     of pregnancy
┌───┴────────┐
+ve, confirms    –ve, consider PUPPP,
pemphigoid       prurigo of pregnancy,
gestationis      pruritic folliculitis of
                 pregnancy
```

flare during or after delivery. Some patients have a mild urticarial during one pregnancy but may have severe blistering during a subsequent pregnancy. In 5–10% women, the disease may occur in a pregnancy, then skip the next pregnancy and recur in a subsequent pregnancy.[19] The disease may recur with menstruation especially during the first few cycles following delivery. A quarter of patients will have flares with subsequent oral contraceptive use.

Treatment

The rarity of PG precludes controlled studies for its treatment. There is general consensus that antihistaminics and topical steroids are ineffective and systemic corticosteroids are the mainstay of therapy. Most patients respond to 0.5 mg/kg prednisolone, some require maintenance throughout pregnancy, others do not. There are anecdotal reports of using dapsone, pyridoxine, cyclosporine, plasmapheresis as alternatives to steroid therapy. Intravenous immunoglobulin is also useful.

REFERENCES

1. Sterling JC Chapter 33: Virus infections In: Rook's Textbook of Dermatology 8th ed. Eds Burns T, Breathnach S, Cox N, Griffiths C. Wiley Blackwell 2010.

2. Sauerbrei A, Wutzler P. Herpes simplex and varicella-zoster virus infections during pregnancy: current concepts of prevention, diagnosis and therapy. Part 1: Herpes simplex virus infections. Med Microbiol Immunol 2007; 196:89–94

3. Brown ZA, Vontver LA, Benedetti J et al. Effects on infants of a first episode of genital herpes during pregnancy. New Engl J Med 1987; 317:1246–51.

4. Prober CG, Sullender WM, Yasukawa LL et al. Low risk of herpes simplex virus infections in neonates exposed to the virus at the time of vaginal delivery to mothers with recurrent genital herpes simplex virus infections. New Engl J Med 1987; 316:240–4.

5. Money D, Steben M, Wong T et al. Guidelines for the management of herpes simplex virus in pregnancy. J Obstet. Gynaecol. Can. June 2008; 30(6):514–26.

6. Pardo J, Yogev Y, Ben-Haroush A et al. Primary herpes simplex virus type 1 gingivostomatitis during the second and third trimester of pregnancy: Foetal and pregnancy outcome. Scand J Infect Dis 2004; 36:179–81.

7. Mercolini F, Verdi F, Eisendle K et al. Congenital disseminated HSV-1 infection in preterm twins after primary gingivostomatitis of the mother: case report and review of the literature. Z Gebertshilfe Neonatol 2014 Dec; 218(6):261–4.

8. Li DK, Raebel MA, Cheetham TC et al. Genital herpes and its treatment in relation to preterm delivery. Am J Epidemiol 2014 Dec; 180(11):1109–17.

9. Ambros-Rudolph CM, Shornick JK Chapter 27: Pregnancy dermatoses In: Dermatology 3rd ed. Eds. Bolognia JL, Jorizzo JL, Schaffer JV Elsevier Saunders.

10. Villota VA, Delgado J, Pachajoa H. Congenital varicella syndrome in a monochorionic-diamniotic twin pregnancy. J Res. Med. Sci.2014 May; 19(5): 474–76.

11. Enders G, Miller E, Cradock-Watson J et al. Consequences of varicella and herpes zoster in pregnancy: Prospective study of 1739 cases. Lancet 1994; 343:1548–51.

12. Mendelson E, Aboudy Y, Smetana Z. Laboratory diagnosis and assessment of congenital viral infections. ReprodToxicol. 2006 May; 21(4):350–82.

13. Shrim A, Koren G, Yudin MH. Management of varicella infection in pregnancy. J ObstetGynecol Can 2012 Mar; 34(3):287–92.

14. Wojnarowska F, Venning VA 40: Immunobullous diseases In: Rook's Textbook of Dermatology 8th ed. Eds. Burns T, Breathnach S, Cox N, Griffiths C. Wiley Blackwell 2010.

15. Matsumoto N, Osada M, Kaneko K et al. Pemphigoid gestationis after spontaneous expulsion of a massive complete hydatidiform mole. Case Rep Obstet Gynaecol 2013;2013:267–268.

16. Djahansouzi S, Nestle-Kraemling C, Dall P et al. Herpes gestationis may present itself as a paraneoplastic syndrome of choriocarcinoma—a case report. Gynecol. Oncol. 2003 May; 89(2): 334–7.

17. Shornick JK, Black MM: Fetal risks in herpes gestationis. J Am AcadDermatol 26:63, 1992.

18. Shornick JK, Black MM: Secondary autoimmune diseases in herpes gestationis (pemphigoid-gestationis). J Am Acad Dermatol 26:563, 1992.

19. Holmes RC et al: Clues to the aetiology and pathogenesis of herpes gestationis. Br J Dermatol1983;109:131.

22

HPV in Pregnancy

Madhuri Mehendale, Reena Wani

HUMAN PAPILLOMAVIRUS

HPV is one of the most common STDs with over 30 types infecting the genital area, High risk types 16 and 18 are associated with dysplasia. Mucocutaneous external genital warts are usually caused by HPV types 6 and 11 but may be caused by intermediate and high oncogenic risk HPV.

The highest rates of genital infection are detected in adults age 18 to 28. Major risk factors to acquiring genital HPV infection include multiple sex partners, younger age at first intercourse and first pregnancy, oral contraceptive use, pregnancy and impairment of cell-mediated immunity.

Controversial data exists on a possible increase in the prevalence of HPV infections during pregnancy. Up to threefold increase in HPV DNA-positive women is seen during the third trimester as compared to non-pregnant controls. Possible reason could be hormonal changes inducing virus transcription and the transient immune-suppression experienced by pregnant women.[1]

Diagnosis

Visual diagnosis can be made by appearance of white or pink verrucous friable growths. However, most cases are subclinical. Screening for cervical cancer in pregnancy with pap smear is standard practice in many countries, and in certain places in India too. Triaging by HPV DNA testing has been suggested as an adjunct to abnormal pap smears and as a possible way to increase screening interval.[2] Papanicolau smear may detect infection in 10–30%. If koilocytosis detected on pap smear, either triaging with HPV DNA testing or colposcopy is warranted. Colposcopy may identify up to 70% infected cases.

The usefulness of DNA technology in the clinical diagnosis of genital warts is not supported by any data. Screening for subclinical HPV infection by DNA or RNA tests is not recommended.[3]

Maternal Risks

Genital warts frequently increase in number and size during pregnancy for reasons unknown. Lesions filling up the vagina or covering the perineum, thus making vaginal delivery or episiotomy difficult.

As HPV infection may be subclinical and multifocal, most women with vulvar lesions also have cervical infection and vice versa

Neonatal Infection

HPV types 6 and 11 often associated with juvenile onset recurrent papillomatosis, is a rare benign neoplasm of the larynx. It can cause hoarseness and respiratory distress in children. Studies differ in their findings of neonatal transmission rates. Conservative estimates suggest the risk approximately 1 in 400. Prolonged rupture of membranes was associated with a two-fold increased risk, but no risk associated with the mode of delivery.

Benefit of cesarean delivery to decrease transmission risk is unknown, and thus it is currently not recommended solely to prevent HPV transmission (Centers for disease Control and Prevention, 2006b).The presence of HPV has been demonstrated in amniotic fluid, placenta and cord blood, thus the fetus is at risk for exposure to the virus prior to delivery.[4]

Management Options[5]

Pre-pregnancy

Some genital warts resolve spontaneously; however, treatment should be considered for expanding genital warts

Identify and Treat Lesions

- Topical therapy (podophyllum resin 10% to 25% antimitotic solution, podofilox 0.5% solution, 5-fluorouracil)
- Ablation
- Removal

Counsel about risks (infectious condition) and use of condoms if partner infected.

Advice that treatment does not eradicate infectivity and all treatments have a 10–40% probability of recurrence.

Implications from cervical smear screening programs:

If pap smear reports ASCUS but no other types of abnormalities
- Consider HPV testing

If pap smear reports ASCUS, and high risk HPV types are detected
- Perform colposcopy, consider biopsy
- Perform pelvic examination, pap smear on a regular basis

Screening for sub-clinical HPV infection is not recommended.

Prenatal

Topical 80%TCA—least expensive, not absorbed systemically, cure rate of 20–30% after single application so weekly repeated till lesion resolved.

Cryotherapy with liquid nitrogen is the first line treatment option, not recommended for use in the vagina because of risk of vaginal perforation and fistula formation.

Electrodiathermy

Laser vaporisation (carbon dioxide)—recurrence rates of 10–14%.

Excision(tangential scissors, excision, curettage)—advantage of elimination in single visit. *Contraindicated preparations in pregnancy:*
- Podophyllum
- Podofilox
- 5-fluorouracil
- Interferon

Counsel about low newborn risk, and about nature of HPV infection in the infant.

Labor and Delivery

Avoid treatment at delivery especially debulking, becuse of risk of hemorrhage, also most lesions regress to some extent after delivery.

Cesarean section may be indicated in women with genital warts obstructing labor or vaginal delivery that would result in excessive bleeding. It is not recommended solely to prevent HPV transmission to the infant.

Postnatal

Maintain vigilance for secondary infection, especially in episiotomy site. Offer Sitz baths.

HPV Vaccine Recommendations[2, 6]

HPV vaccine can be administered when a female patient is breastfeeding. HPV vaccine is not recommended during pregnancy. The practitioner should inquire about pregnancy in sexually active female patients, but a pregnancy test is not required before starting the immunization series. If a vaccine recipient becomes pregnant, subsequent doses should be postponed until completion of the pregnancy. It is recommended that women who become pregnant while receiving HPV vaccine be reported to registries that have been developed to record data on outcomes (HPV2: 1-888-452-9622; PV4:1-800-986-8999).

Despite vaccination, standard screening for cervical cancer (i.e. Papanicolaou testing) should continue to be conducted in women who have received HPV vaccine. Administration of HPV vaccine does not change current counselling recommendations for use of barrier methods for the prevention of HPV and other sexually transmitted infections as well as discussion about healthy choices about sexual activity, including condoms and abstinence.

REFERENCES

1. Rando RF, Lindhiem S, Hasty L, et al: Increased frequency of detection of human papillomavirus DNA in exfoliated cervical cells during pregnancy. Am J Obstet Gynecol 1989;161:50–54.

2. Triple A Guideline: ACS, ASCCP, American Society for Clinical Pathology CA Cancer J Clinics March 2012.

3. Centers for Disease Control: Sexually transmitted disease guidelines. MMWR 2002;51:1–80.

4. Ambruster-Moraes E, et al. Presence of human papillomavirus DNA in amniotic fluids of pregnant women with cervical lesions. Gynecol Oncol 1994;54: 152–158.

5. David K. James: High risk Pregnancy, Third Edition, Chapter 31;663–664.

6. HPV Vaccine Recommendations. AAP Committee on Infectious Diseases. Pediatrics 2012;129;602; originally published online February 27, 2012; DOI: 10.1542/peds.2011–3865.

23

HIV in Pregnancy—Latest Guidelines

Sarita Agrawal, Shreya Goenka

INTRODUCTION

NACP (National AIDS Control Programme) was launched in 1992 and has evolved through the decades as NACP II in 1999, NACP III in 2007 and NACP IV in 2012 to control Human Immunodeficiency Virus (HIV) and Acquired Immunodeficiency Syndrome (AIDS) changing from a national response to a more decentralised method by involving NGOs and networks of People Living with HIV(PLHIV). The adult (15–49 age group) HIV prevalence at national level has continued its steady decline from estimated level of 0.41% in 2001 to 0.27% in 2011.[1] But still, India is estimated to have the third highest number of estimated people living with HIV / AIDS, after South Africa and Nigeria (UNAIDS Report on the Global AIDS epidemic 2010). Women constitute 39 % of the PLHIV in India and children below 15 years-constitute 7%.[2] Without any intervention the risk of vertical transfer is 20 to 45%.[2]

Global evidences show that a single dose Nevirapine (SD-NVP) although effective, offers partial protection, i.e does not prevent transmission in antenatal period and during breastfeeding and increases the risk of co-resistance to NVP and Efavirenz (NNRTIs). Hence, multiple drug ARV regimens starting early in pregnancy and continuing until cessation of breastfeeding have potential to reduce the transmission to less than 5%. Based upon these evidences the guidelines for ART (Anti Retroviral Therapy) for PPTCT (Prevention Of Parent to Child Transmission) are revised in the year 2013.

WHO NEW GUIDELINES

WHO new guidelines (June 2013) recommend two options:[3]

1. Providing lifelong ART to all the pregnant and breastfeeding women with HIV regardless of CD4 count or clinical stage OR

2. Providing ART for pregnant and breast-feeding women living with HIV during mother-to-child transmission risk period. Short-term ARV prophylaxis to prevent MTCT during pregnancy, delivery and breastfeeding for HIV-infected women not in need of treatment (i.e CD4 counts less than > 350/mm[3] or clinical stage < 3 or 4). Then continuing life long ART for those women eligible for their own health.

NEW GUIDELINES IN INDIA

Depending on these guidelines, Department of AIDS Control (DAC) India and NACO (National Aids Control Organisation) has decided to opt for the first option of triple drug ART to all pregnant and breastfeeding women regardless of CD4 count and clinical staging. Preferred regimen is TDF + 3TC + EFZ. (Tenofovir + Lamivudine + Efavirenz)

Advantages of this regimen are:
1. Maximises coverage.

2. Avoids stopping and starting drugs with repeat pregnancies.
3. Provide early protection against Mother-to-child Transmission (MTCT) in future pregnancies.
4. Avoids drug resistance.

These guidelines were implemented across the country since 1st January 2014.[2]

GOALS OF NATIONAL PPTCT PROGRAMME IN INDIA

1. Primary prevention of HIV, especially among women in child-bearing age.
2. Integration of PPTCT interventions with general health services.
3. Strengthening post-natal care of the HIV-infected mother and her exposed infant.
4. Provide the essential package of PPTCT services.

THE ESSENTIAL PACKAGE OF SERVICES UNDER THE PPTCT PROGRAMME

1. Routine offer of HIV counselling (group/individual counselling) and testing to all pregnant women attending antenatal care, with 'opt out' option.

2. Provide ART to all HIV infected pregnant women regardless of WHO staging and CD4 count results. Preferred regimen is TDF+3TC+ EFV.
3. Provision of care for associated conditions like STI/RTI, TB and other Opportunistic Infections (OIs).
4. Promote institutional delivery for all HIV infected pregnant women (ANMs/ASHAs, Community workers to accompany to institutions).
5. Provide counselling and support for initiation of exclusive breastfeeds within an hour of delivery as the preferred option and continue for 6 months. After 6 months, complementary feeding should be given along with breastfeeds. A small number of babies born to HIV infected mothers who have serious illness or have died and a few reluctant mothers (who at their own risk despite counselling) may decide not to breastfeed but adopt exclusive replacement feeding (ERF) may be given. Ensure involvement of spouse and other family members and move from an "ANC centric" to a "Family centric" approach (Fig. 23.1).

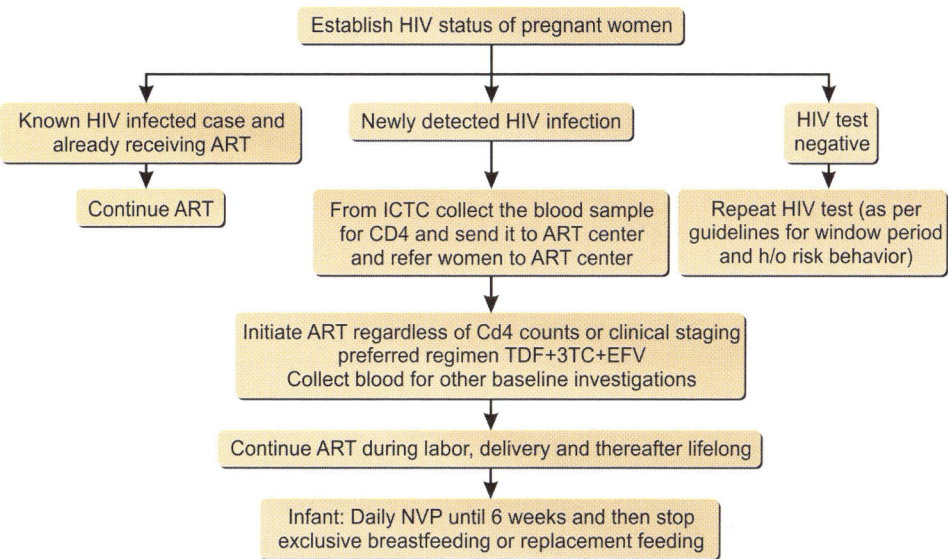

Fig. 23.1: Summary of the technical guidelines and options for the more efficacious PPTCT regimen[2]

6. Provide antiretroviral prophylaxis to infants from birth up to a minimum period of 6 weeks.
7. Ensure initiation of co-trimoxazole Prophylactic Therapy (CPT) and Early Infant Diagnosis (EID) using HIV DNA PCR at 6 weeks of age onwards as per the EID guidelines.
8. Ensure involvement of spouse and other family members and to move from an "ANC centric" to a "Family centric" approach.

First and foremost step is to determine the HIV status of the pregnant woman.

PROCESS OF HIV SCREENING

When to do: All ANC preferably at the first visit. Repeat testing after 6 months after the most recent risk event to cover the window period.

Patient who comes direct-in-labor: Single rapid test to be performed in labor room itself and if found positive ART should be started.

Patient who comes in the postpartum period: Single rapid test is done first and if positive start ART. Provide 6 weeks supply of infant syrup NVP prophylaxis at ICTCs for all HIV exposed babies (3 bottles of Sy NVP:25 ml) Arrange for monthly follow-up of the infants. Such mothers have to be on lifelong ART.

Screen for TB as risk of active TB is 10 times more in HIV pregnant women than in normal population.[4] Active TB can contribute to prematurity, LBW (Low Birth Weight), and perinatal TB among infants. A recent study in India found that TB increases the mother-to-child transmission by 2.5 times.[4]

The list of the screening assays for HIV testing is given below:
1. ELISA (2–3 hours)
2. Rapid tests (minutes)
   - Dot blot assays (immunoconcentration, vertical flow of reagents)
   - Particle agglutination .
   - HIV spot and comb tests.
   - Immunochromatography (lateral flow of reagents).
   - Dipstick and comb assays (based on ELISA technology) (Fig. 23.2)

STEPS FOR ANTENATAL CARE IN HIV POSITIVE WOMEN

1. Link with ART centre
2. WHO clinical staging
3. Screening for TB.
4. Look for and treat STIs.
5. Baseline CD4 counts and repeat every 6 months
6. Start Co-trimoxazole (CPT) if CD4 count ≤ 250 cells/mm^3 and then it is to be continued throughout pregnancy, delivery and breastfeeding in a dose of double strength 1 tab daily. This is done to prevent opportunistic infections like Toxoplasmosis, *Pneumocystis pneumoniae*, diarrhea and other bacterial infections.
7. Counsel for institutional delivery, adherence to ART center, regular antenatal check up.
8. Exclusive breastfeeding and no mixed feeding < 6 months infant.
9. Start ART as soon as possible even in first trimester. Preferred treatment is once daily dose combination of Tenofovir (TDF) (300 mg) + Lamivudine (3TC) (300 mg) + Efavirenz (EFV) (600 mg) if there is no prior exposure to NNRTIs at any gestational age.
10. Alternate first line regimen includes AZT (Zidovudine)
    - AZT + 3TC + EFV
    - AZT +3TC + NVP
    - TDF + 3TC + NVP
11. In patients with previous exposure to sd-NVP or EFV, require protease inhibitors
    - TDF + 3TC + LPV/r (Lopinavir/Ritonavir)
    - Dose will be TDF + 3TC(1 tablet daily) + LPV (200 mg)/r(50 mg)(2 tablets BD)
12. Pregnant women already receiving ART should continue the same regimen.

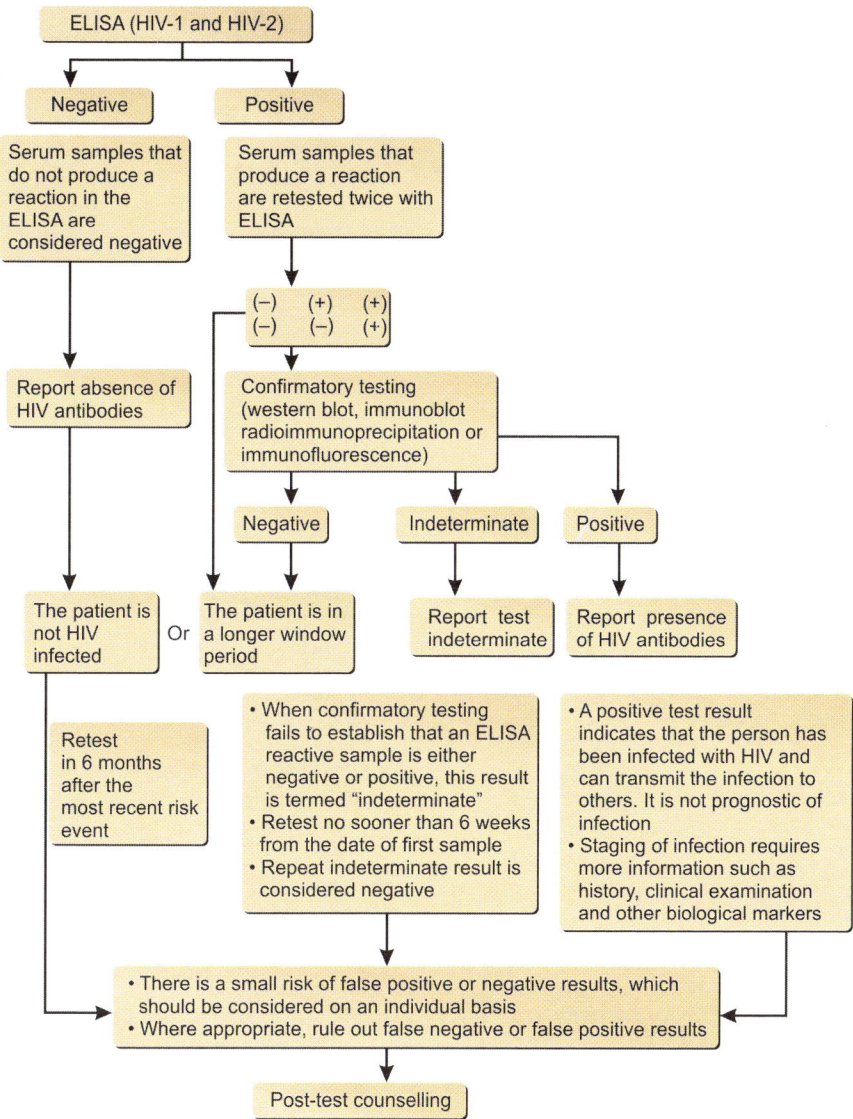

Fig. 23.2: Post-test counselling

MANAGEMENT OF HEI (HIV EXPOSED INFANTS)

1. Syrup Nevirapine for the newborn infant from birth till 6 weeks of age (minimum) to be started within 12 hrs of birth.

2. If the duration of mothers ART is less than 6 months (optimal duration for viral suppression), the dose of NVP should be increased to 12 weeks.

3. The above criteria (2) is only for breastfeeding infants and not for replacement feeding infants.

4. CPT (Co-trimoxazole prophylactic Treatment) is initiated and continued till 18 months or until the confirmatory test of the baby is done using all three Rapid Antibody Tests. If the baby tests positive, the CPT is continued along with pediatric ART (Table 23.1).

Table 23.1: Clinical and laboratory monitoring of pregnant women receiving ART							
Assessment	Baseline	2 weeks	4 weeks	8 weeks	12 weeks	Every 6 months	Comment
Clinical evaluation	√	√	√	√	√	√	Every month
Adherence counselling	√	√	√	√	√	√	Every month
Weight	√	√	√	√	√	√	Every month
Hemoglobin	√	√	√	√	√	√	Recheck at 28–32 wks
ALT	√	√	X	X	X	√	As and when required
Urinalysis	√					√	
CD4	√					√	
Blood urea/ serum creatinine	√					√	Esp. in TDF regimen
Blood grouping	√						
HBV and HCV screening	√						
RPR/VDRL	√						
Blood sugar	√						
Lipid profile*	√						

*Lipid profile and blood sugar at baseline, at 6 months and one year, if started on LPV/r regimen.

Table 23.2: Dosage schedule and common side effects with ARV drugs			
	Name of ARV	Dose	Side-effects
1	Tenofovir TDF	300 mg once daily	Nephrotoxicity, hyperphosphatemia
2	Lamivudine (3TC)	300 mg once daily	Very few side effects: Hypersensitivity
3	Efavirenz	600 mg once daily	Neuro-psychiatric symptoms
4	Lopinavir (LPV/r)	200/50 mg twice daily	
		2 tabs daily	Gastrointestinal disturbance, glucose intolerance, lipo-dystrophy and hyperlipidemia.

5. Recommended daily dose of Co-trimoxazole:
   - For infants below 6 months or < 5 kg (100 mg sulfamethoxazole/20 mg trimethoprim)
   - For children 6 months–5 years or 5–15 kg (200 mg/40 mg)
   - For children 6–14 years old or 15–30 kg (400 mg/80 mg)
   - For anyone over 14 years or >30 kg (800 mg/160 mg)

Cotrimoxazole suspension contains 200 mg/40 mg per 5 ml of syrup. Single strength tablets contain 400 mg/80 mg, double strength tablet twice that. It is possible to divide the tablets for children and infants (Table 23.2).

6. Exclusive breastfeeds up to 6 months. Complementary feeds after 6 months up to 1 year. Breastfeeding is to be continued up to 1 year. HIV positive babies who receive Paediatric ART should continue breastfeeding up to 2 years.

7. Breastfeeding should not be stopped abruptly. Stop gradually over 1 month.

8. Mixed feeding is breastfeeding with replacement feeding. Mixed feeding is not recommended as this causes gastric mucosal abrasion that facilitate the entry of HIV virus.

9. If replacement feeding is chosen it should be affordable, feasible, acceptable, safe and sustainable (AFASS criteria should be fulfilled).

10. Infant testing is done at 6 weeks by dry blood spot (DBS) test.
   - If positive, WBS (whole blood sample).
   - If rapid test is negative, repeat test at 6 months,12 months and 6 weeks after cessation of breastfeeds.
   - Final diagnosis at 18 months using 3 antibody tests.

11. If mother interrupts ART while breast-feeding (due to toxicity, stock-outs or refusal to continue), continue syrup NVP until 6 weeks after maternal ART is restarted or until 1 week after breast-feeding has ended.

12. All babies detected to be positive are given pediatric ART irrespective of CD4 counts.

13. Arrange for monthly follow-ups for babies in the first year and thereafter every 3 months irrespective of feeding method.

INTERVENTIONS IN WOMEN DIAGNOSED WITH HIV IN LABOR (DIRECT IN LABOR) AND POSTPARTUM

There is a significant percentage of women with unknown HIV status who directly present in active labor for delivery. They should also be offered routine screening of HIV with opt-out option as per national guidelines. Screening using whole blood finger prick test should be undertaken.

Pregnant women who are found to be positive:

- Initiate on ART (TDF + 3TC + EFV) immediately.
- Next day counsellor visits patients.
- Counsel about exclusive breastfeeding or exclusive replacement feeding.
- Confirm with 3 rapid antibody tests.
- Lab technician should collect blood sample for CD4 test and take it to the laboratory and bring back the report with 1 month ART.
- All infants should receive daily NVP prophylaxis for 6 weeks or more as per guidelines. Daily NVP prophylaxis should be started even if more than 72 hours have passed since birth. At 6 weeks EID should be carried out. CPT initiation and continue until baby is 18 months older and longer if baby tested positive (Table 23.3).

WOMEN REPORTING POSTPARTUM

HIV testing is to be done and if found positive triple drug ART is started along with infant prophylaxis with syrup Nevirapine.

PREGNANT WOMEN WITH HIV 2 INFECTION

HIV 2 also progresses to AIDS though at a slower rate. It has the same modes of transmission but has been shown to be less transmissible from mother to child (transmission risk 0–4%).

NNRTI like NVP and EFV are not effective against HIV 2 infection, so treat with 2 NRTIs + LPV/r. Prophylaxis with AZT (instead of syp NVP) to be given to babies in mothers with HIV 2 (Table 23.4).

If a pregnant woman is detected with both infections, then she is given standard first ART

Table 23.3: Dose and duration of infant daily NVP prophylaxis			
Birth weight	*NVP daily dose (mg)*	*NVP daily dose in ml*	*Duration*
Birth weight <2000 gm	2 mg/kg once daily	0.2 ml/kg/day	Up to 6 weeks
2000–2500 gm	10 mg once daily	1 ml once daily	
>2500 gm	15 mg once daily	1.5 ml once daily	

Table 23.4: Dose of AZT

Birth wt.	AZT Daily Dosage in mg	AZT Daily Dosage in ml	Duration
<2000 gm	5 mg/kg twice daily	0.5 ml twice daily	6 weeks
<2500 gm	10 mg/kg twice daily	1 ml/kg twice daily	6 weeks
>2500 gm	15 mg/kg twice daily	1.5 ml twice daily	6 weeks

regimen (TDF + 3TC + EFV) recommended for women with HIV 1.

CESAREAN SECTION

Cesarean section is not routinely recommended for prevention of mother to child transmission and done only if there is an obstetric indication for the same. It is scheduled at 38 wks or before rupture of membranes.

- For planned cesarean, ART should be given prior to the operation.
- Women on lifelong ART should continue their standard ART regimen.
- In emergency cases ensure that women receive ART prior to the procedure and continue thereafter.
- They should receive standard perioperative antibiotics. Complications of cesarean section is higher in women with HIV, with the most frequently reported complication being postpartum fever.
- Use of safe surgical practices during cesarean section:
  1. Dry hemostatic techniques to minimize bleeding, i.e. good observation and follow surgical planes during dissection, judicious use of electro-cautery.
  2. Senior obstetrician should perform it.
  3. Cord should clamped as early as possible.
  4. Avoid manual removal of placenta.
  5. Round tip blunt needle to be used.
  6. Do not use fingers to hold the needle.
  7. Hold containers to transfer sharps.
  8. For disposal of tissues and placenta standard waste disposal management guidelines should be followed.

SAFER DELIVERY TECHNIQUES

Mother-to-child transmission is increased by the prolonged rupture of membranes, repeated P/V examinations, assisted instrumental deliveries, episiotomy and prematurity. Hence observe:

- Standard Universal Work precautions (UWP).
- Do not rupture membranes artificially (keep membranes intact as long as possible)
- Minimal vaginal examinations.
- Avoid instrumental deliveries and invasive procedures like fetal blood sampling.
- If required low outlet forceps is preferred to ventouse, as it is related with lower rate of fetal trauma than ventouse.
- Avoid routine episiotomy as far as possible.
- Early cord clamping.
- Suctioning the newborn with nasogastric tube should be avoided unless there is meconium staining of the liquor.

POSTPARTUM PERIOD

The postpartum period is especially important for:

- Counselling regarding continuation of life long therapy.
- Counsel about proper diet.
- Counsel regarding exclusive breastfeeding or replacement feeding and weaning after 6 months. To continue breast feeding till 1 year in negative babies and till two years in EID positive babies.
- She should be taught how to give the medication using dropper or syringe.
- To look out for other postpartum complications.

- To look out for postpartum depression which may be the cause for discontinuing ART especially infant NVP.[5]
- To counsel about contraceptive methods like condoms, IUD and NSV.
- To follow up in ART clinic at 6 weeks postpartum which would coincide with the infant's first vaccination.

ESSENTIAL GYNEC CARE OF HIV POSITIVE WOMEN

Women infected with HIV are at higher risk of developing cervical dysplasia leading to cervical cancer. The Human Papillomavirus (HPV) infection is more common in HIV infected pregnant women, particularly Geno types 16, 18 and others incriminated to be carcinogenic being 31, 33, 35, 39, 45, 51, 52, 56, 58, 59 and 68 more incriminated to cause cervical cancer. In the National ART Guidelines for adults and adolescents, cervical screening, e.g. pap smear or trichloro-acetic acid screening of the cervix should be done annually for all HIV infected pregnant women.

CONTRACEPTION

Dual protection with consistent condom use is important.[6] Dual protection refers to simultaneous protection against both unplanned pregnancy and STIs and HIV by using condoms together with another effective method of contraception, including emergency contraception.

Available forms of contraception for HIV infected pregnant women include:

Hormonal contraception is safe in women living with HIV whose CD4 count is > 350 cells/mm³. These may be either:

- Oral contraceptives
- Depot medroxyprogesterone acetate (DMPA)

DMPA is safe to use in women living with HIV as well as those on ART. There is no hormone–drug interaction with several ARV drugs commonly used such as NVP, EFV and Nelfinavir.

Adherence to oral contraception needs to be counselled. In women taking ART for their own health, they should be assessed for oral contraception use according to the WHO Medical Eligibility Criteria[7] for Contraceptive Use guidelines. There may be hormone–drug interactions which need dosing to be adjusted or an alternative contraception to be used.

RITONAVIR/NEVIRAPINE

- Combined oral contraception pills are generally not recommended, due to the potentially decreased efficacy of the contraception.
- Efavirenz
- Women taking EFV may be able to take combined oral contraception without loss of contraceptive efficacy
- *NRTI such as AZT and TDF:* Women taking AZT and TDF may take combined oral contraception without loss of contraceptive efficacy

Lactational Amenorrhoea Method (LAM) does not protect against STIs, pregnancy and HIV. Correct and consistent condom use should be adopted at every sexual encounter.

Male sterilization (NSV): Males should be motivated at every mother–baby pair follow-up visit to undergo sterilization. No Scalpel Vasectomy (NSV) when the baby attains 18 months/2 years of age (at 18 months confirmatory test, irrespective of the baby's HIV status). However, after NSV operation, male should continue to use a condom at every sexual encounter.[7]

Intra-Uterine Contraceptive Device (IUCD) is a good contraceptive inserted within 48 hrs of delivery. IUCD[8] Copper T 380A is recommended by MoHFW as a long term reversible method of contraception up to 10 years.

REFERENCES

1. National Guidelines for Prevention Of Parent to Child Transmission of HIV, June 2013. http://www.naco.gov.in/upload/Publication/Basic%20Services/National% 20 Guidelines%20 for%20PPTCT_01_05_2013.pdf

2. National Guidelines For Prevention Of Parent to child Transmission, Dec 2013 page 12. http://naco.gov.in/upload/NACP%20-%20IV/18022014%20BSD/National_Guidelines_for_PPTCT.pdf

3. World Health Organisation, Consolidated guidelines on the use of Antiretroviral drugs for treating and preventing HIV infection, recommendation for Public Health Approach, June 2013. http://www.who.int/hiv/pub/mtct/PMTCTfactsheet/en/

4. Maternal Tuberculosis: A Risk Factor for Mother-to-Child-Transmission of Human Immuno-deficiency virus. Gupta A, Bhosale R, Kinikar A, et al for the Six Week Extended-Dose Nevirapine (SWEN) India Study Team. JID 2011:203(3), 358–63 (1 February). http://www.researchgate.net/publication/49731399_Maternal_tuberculosis_a_risk_factor_for_mother-to-child_transmission_of_human_ immunodeficiency_virus

5. Postpartum psychiatric care in India: The need for integration and innovation. Prabha S Chandra. World Psychiatry. 2004 June; 3(2): 99–100.

6. Sexual and reproductive health of women living with HIV/AIDS Guidelines on care, treatment and support for women living with HIV/AIDS and their children in resource-constrained settings. WHO/UNFPA 2006.

7. Medical Eligibility Criteria for Contraceptive Use. 4th edition. WHO 2009. http://www.who.int/reproductivehealth/publications/family_planning.

8. IUCD Reference manual for Medical Officers 2013. Family Planning Division. MoHFW. http://www.nrhmtn.gov.in/modules/IUCD_Reference_Manual_for_MOs_and_Nursing_Personne_-Final-Sept_2013.pdf

24

TORCH Infections and Pregnancy

Rashmi G Jalvee, Reena Wani

TORCH infections or Toxoplasmosis, Others (syphilis, hepatitis, zoster), Rubella, Cytomegalovirus and Herpes simplex, are a group of maternal infections that have a few maternal symptoms, lack effective therapy and can have major consequences for the fetus. Concerns with congenital infections are focused on the possible vertical transmission of these infections to the fetus, which may lead to various forms of malformations, neurodevelopmental delay and long term childhood consequences. These may manifest as febrile illness in pregnancy.

All these infections have their own causative agent and generally spread through poor hygienic conditions, contaminated blood, water and soil and airborne respiratory droplet.

TOXOPLASMOSIS

Causative Organism

Toxoplasmosis is a benign anthropozoonosis, caused by *Toxoplasma gondii* (*T. gondii*), an obligate intracellular protozoan. Its life cycle

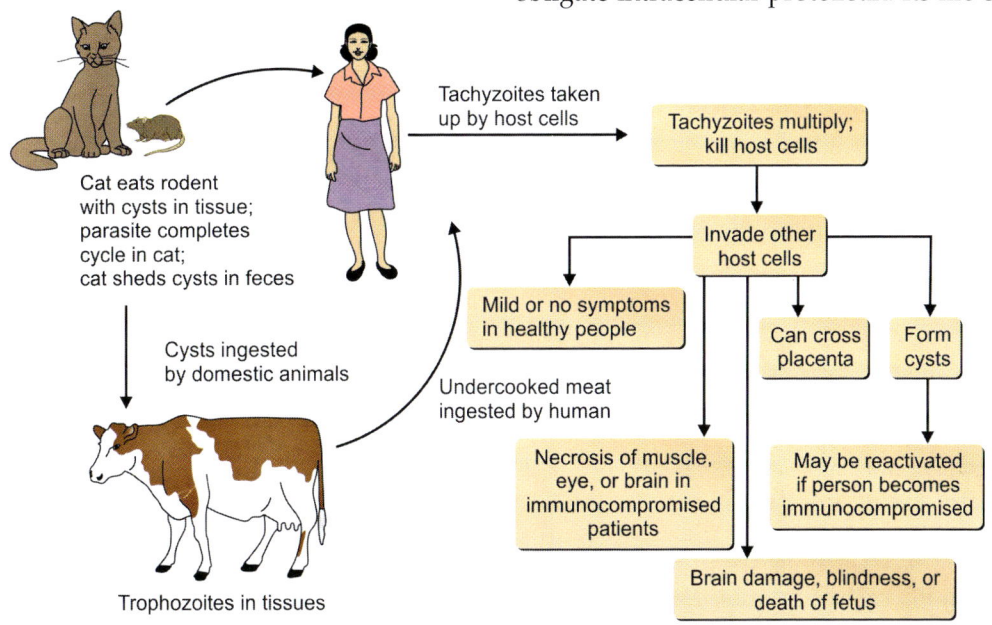

Fig. 24.1: Mode of infection

includes sexual reproduction in the definitive host, the cat, and asexual division in intermediate hosts which include man, birds and rodents.[1]

Mode of Infection

The human infection may be acquired by ingestion of oocysts excreted by cats and contaminating soil or water, or by eating tissue cysts that remain viable in undercooked meat of infected animals.[2] The organism is carried by wild rodents and cats and in its oocyst form can persist for extended periods in soil (Fig. 24.1).

Clinical Manifestations

Primary infection is often asymptomatic. Even when symptoms do occur, they are nonspecific, or appear as a viral syndrome, such as fever, malaise and lymphadenopathy (which involves the posterior cervical chain). Immunosuppression facilitates development of severe disease and can cause chorioretinitis and encephalitis.

Fetal Transmission

Maternal infection can affect the fetus in all trimesters but the severity of fetal damage is higher in the first and the second trimester than in the third. Following primary infection during pregnancy, fetal transmission is 25% in the first trimester (75% severely affected), 50% in the second trimester (55% severely affected) and 65% after 28 weeks (<5% severely affected).

Fetal Sequelae

- Abortions
- CNS manifestations like hydrocephalus, microcephaly, intra-cerebral calcification and ventriculomegaly.
- Ocular manifestations like cataract, chorioretinitis and blindness
- Newborn may also have learning disabilities, seizures, spasticity.
- Anemia, rash, hepatosplenomegaly or jaundice.

Diagnosis

Most commonly, the diagnosis is not made in the mother until abnormalities are seen on ultrasound or an affected child is born. Occasionally, suspicion is engendered by a mononucleosis-like syndrome, especially if the circumstances suggest it (ingestion of raw meat or contact with cats).

The most common method of diagnosis is by means of serology. Both IgM and IgG antibodies generally appear 1–2 weeks after the initial infection (Fig. 24.2).

The problem in diagnosis is to differentiate acute infection from a residual titer representing a past infection. IgM antibodies may persist for years in healthy individuals. Positive IgG and IgM titers do not necessarily indicate a recent infection. In such a case, the test result must be confirmed in a reference laboratory, which will run additional tests to determine the time of infection, viz. Sabin-Feldman test, IgM-IFA, IgM ELISA and IgG avidity test.

IgG avidity test is an important test because the strength of antibody binding to the parasite increases approximately 5 months

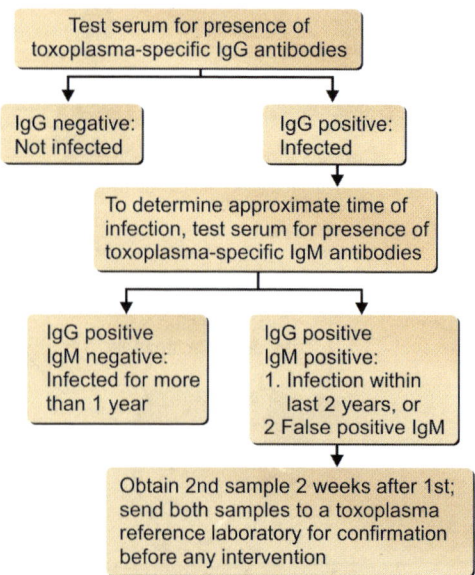

Fig. 24.2: Serum test

after primary infection. In case of positive IgM antibodies and unknown timing of infection, high avidity can rule out primary infection early in pregnancy in around 75% of patients.

If serologic evidence is suggestive of primary infection, the next step is to confirm or rule out fetal infection. Chorionic villus sampling, amniocentesis and cordocentesis with analysis of fetal blood have all been used. A number of techniques have been used to evaluate these specimens, including IgM testing, tissue culture and mouse inoculation. More recently, a polymerase chain reaction (PCR) method has proved both accurate and rapid.[3] Ultrasound findings of hydrocephaly, intracranial calcifications, or hydrops may provide indirect evidence of congenital *Toxoplasma* infection.[4]

If the diagnosis is suspected at delivery, it can be confirmed by histologic evaluation of the placenta, which must be promptly fixed in formalin.

The diagnosis in the newborn is suspected on the basis of clinical findings or from a diagnosis established in the mother. It is confirmed by a positive specific IgM test or a persistent or rising IgG titer, indicating it is of neonatal and not maternal origin.

A summary of diagnosis of toxoplasma infection is shown in Fig. 24.3.[5]

Treatment

Therapy is generally not required for the mother because most adults, if immunologically intact, recover spontaneously.

When the diagnosis of acute *Toxoplasma* infection is established during pregnancy and ideally confirmed in the fetus, there are two management options:

- *Termination of pregnancy:* As the fetal consequences are severe, especially if infection occurs in the first trimester.
- *Treat the mother:* In an effort to reduce the incidence and severity of vertical transmission.

In pregnant women with suspected or confirmed to have acquired toxoplasmosis infection:

Table 24.1: Drug dosages			
	Medication	*Dosage*	*Duration of therapy*
Pregnant women with suspected or documented infection (<18 wks gestation)	Spiramycin	1 g (3 million units) 8 hrly (for a total of 3 g/ 9 million U per day)	Treatment should be continued until delivery in women with low suspicion of fetal infection or those with documented negative results of amniotic fluid PCR or negative findings on ultrasound on follow up
Pregnant women with suspected or documented infection (>18 wks gestation)	Pyrimethamine	Loading dose 100 mg per day in 2 divided doses for 2 days, then 50 mg/day	Until birth
	Sulphadiazine	Loading dose 75 mg/kg/day in 2 divided doses (max 4 g/day) for 2 days, then 100 mg/kg/day in 2 divided doses (max 4 g/day)	Until birth
	Leucovorin	10–20 mg/day	During and after 1 week after pyrimethamine therapy

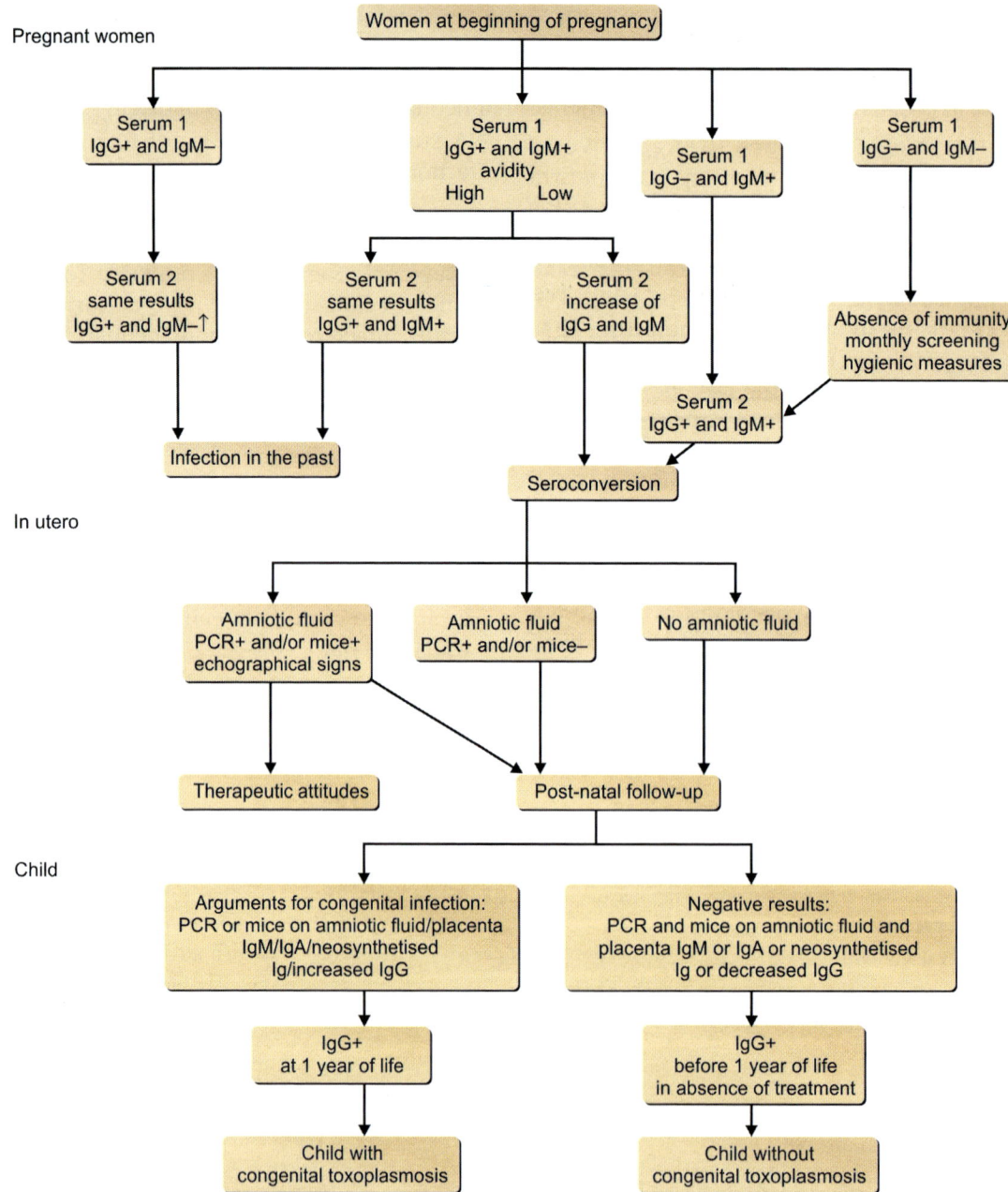

Fig. 24.3: Diagnosis of toxoplasma infection

- **< 18 weeks of gestation:** Spiramycin to be started

  To do an ultrasound and an amniotic fluid PCR at >18 weeks of gestation or soon thereafter as feasible

  - PCR negative and ultrasound negative: to continue spiramycin
  - PCR positive and/or ultrasound positive: pyrimethamine + sulfadiazine +folinic acid

- **> 18 weeks of gestation:** Pyrimethamine + Sulfadiazine + Folinic acid

To do an ultrasound and an amniotic fluid PCR at >18 weeks of gestation or soon thereafter as feasible

- PCR negative and ultrasound negative: consider switching to spiramycin or continue pyrimethamine + sulfadiazine +folinic acid
- PCR positive and/or ultrasound positive: pyrimethamine + sulfadiazine + folinic acid

The details of the drug doses[6] are given in Table 24.1.

Therapy for the symptomatic newborn is accomplished with the same drugs; however, several courses are often necessary. Infants with no symptoms should be treated only if the specific IgM test is positive or if IgG is stable or rising. Isolation is not necessary.

Prevention

The obvious means of prevention of congenital toxoplasmosis are preventing infection during pregnancy and detecting infection during pregnancy to provide early treatment.

Important infection avoidance measures include:

- Avoid eating raw or undercooked meat
- Wash fruits and vegetables carefully
- Wear gloves and thoroughly washing hands after handling soil and gardening
- Avoid cat faeces in cat litter or in soil.

RUBELLA

Causative Organism

Rubella or German measles is caused by a single stranded RNA virus which belongs to the Togaviridae family. The virus consists of an envelope and an icosahedral capsid.

Mode of Infection

The virus is highly contagious and is transmitted through direct contact or airborne droplets from the respiratory system. Its incubation period is about 2–3 weeks. The virus enters the upper respitatory tract, multiplies, invades the cervical lymph nodes and after 7–10 days enters the blood stream and has widespread dissemination. The period of infectivity is 7 days before and 7 days after the appearance of rash.

Clinical Manifestations

Majority of infected individuals are symptomatic and develop symptoms such as fever, malaise, maculopapular rash, post-auricular lymphadenopathy, arthralgia and conjunctivitis. The rash spreads from the face to the trunk and lastly to the extremities and lasts for 3 days. Other manifestations include Forchheimer's spots on the soft palate, Kopliks spots on the buccal mucosa, rubelliform rash (1–3 mm in diameter) and rarely arthritis, encephalitis, thrombocytopenia, hemorrhagic manifestations, neuritis, orchitis, etc.

Fetal Transmission

Rubella virus enters into mother's body, spreads through blood, placenta and infects the fetus. The fetus is at risk of congenital rubella syndrome only during primary infection (Table 24.2). The earlier the maternal infection, the greater is the fetal infection and damage.

Fetal Sequelae

The virus is severely fetopathic in the first trimester and may result in spontaneous abortion. The classical triad of congenital reubella syndrome includes eye, ear and heart

Table 24.2: Fetal transmission		
Gestation (weeks)	Fetal infection (%)	Fetal affection or damage (%)
4–12	>80	>80
12–16	55	20–25
>16	45	Very low risk

abnormalities along with other manifestations:

- *Ocular:* Cataracts, glaucoma, microphthalmia, retinopathy.
- *Cardiac:* Patent ductus arteriosus, pulmonary arterial stenosis, pulmonary valvular stenosis.
- *Auditory:* Sensorineural deafness which is progressive and bilateral.
- *CNS:* Microcephaly, mental retardation.
- *Lung:* Interstitial pneumonitis
- *Hepatic:* Hepatitis, hepatosplenomegaly, jaundice
- *Endocrine:* Diabetes, thyroid dysfunction, growth hormone deficiency
- *Skin:* Blueberry muffin spots, chronic rubelliform rash.

When rubella occurs in the second trimester, the effects are less severe; if it occurs in the third trimester, there may be no obvious effects, except for a positive IgM antibody test in the cord blood. Unfortunately, however, the viral genome tends to remain latent in neural tissue. The newborn with congenital rubella sheds virus for up to 1 year and consequently is an infectious hazard to healthcare personnel. The placenta is also a source of virus.

Diagnosis

Serological testing of the mother is the primary mode of diagnosis. Seroconversion in paired samples is indicative of infection (IgG immunoglobulin remains positive for life).The cornerstone for the assessment of maternal immunity is serological tesing. The most widely used test is the hemagglutination-inhibition test.

The algorithm for diagnosis of rubella is given in Fig. 24.4.

Treatment

Treatment of the mother who has rubella is limited to symptomatic measures because the

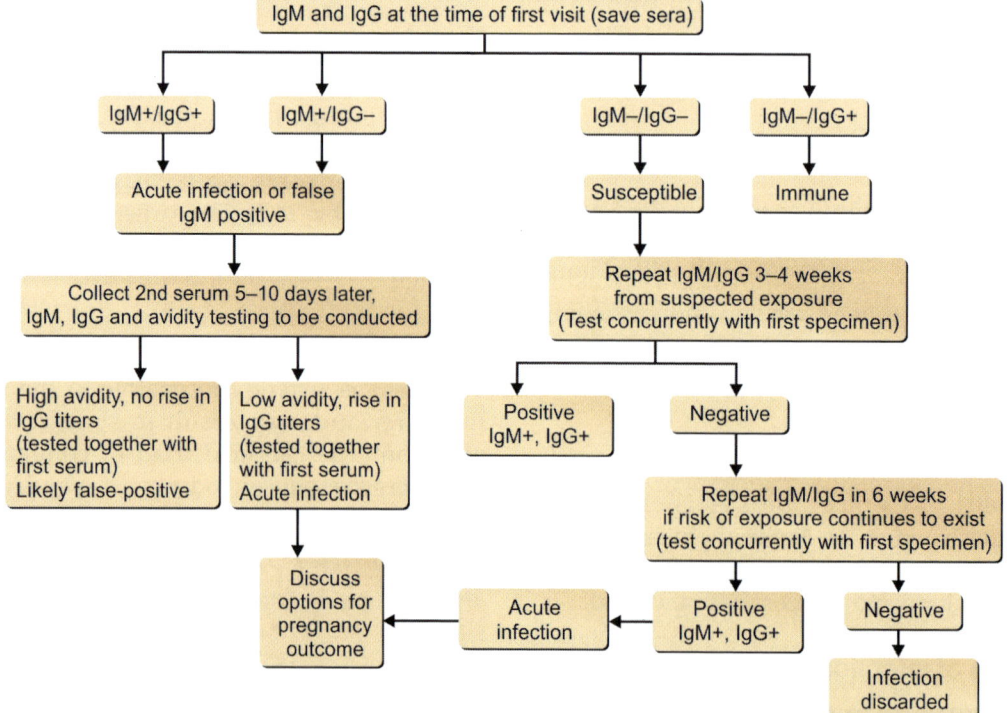

Fig. 24.4: Diagnosis of Rubella

illness is not a serious one. Essentially, then, appropriate management for the gravida with rubella is to provide the information necessary for her to make a considered decision regarding the continuation of the pregnancy. If the pregnant woman is known to be immune by prior testing, only reassurance is needed.

Rubella Vaccine

With the development of rubella vaccine, there is now at least the theoretical possibility for preventing congenital rubella. Because natural immunity protects 80–90% of women in the reproductive age group, the remainder might be covered by childhood immunization. Unfortunately, this strategy has not proved effective because a significant number of those immunized may lose detectable antibody in 5–10 years. Although it is still recommended that all children be immunized (at about 15 months of age), women must be retested when they reach childbearing age and vaccinated again if antibody is not detected. This must be done when the woman is not pregnant and will not conceive for at least one cycle. As the fetal risks of the vaccine virus appear to be considerably less than those of the wild virus,[7] there is no reason to recommend pregnancy termination for women inadvertently vaccinated during pregnancy. An alternative time for the vaccination of susceptible women is immediately postpartum, when conception is less likely. Breastfeeding is not contra-indicated for the vaccinated mother. Patients should be tested for immunity before vaccination, and because there is a 5% failure to develop antibody, follow-up titers should be done in 6–12 weeks. Revaccination is indicated if no titer has developed. Complications are not common, the most frequent being a transient arthralgia.

CYTOMEGALOVIRUS

Cytomegalovirus is the most frequent of the TORCH infections affecting the newborn. It is the most common cause of congenital hearing loss and neurological impairment.

Causative Organism

CMV is an icosahedral, enveloped, double stranded DNA virus that is part of the human herpes virus family. As with other members of this family, it has the ability to establish latency and reactivate at a later time.

Mode of Infection

CMV is transmitted by contact with infected blood, saliva, urine or by sexual contact. The incubation period is 30–60 days. CMV is isolated from the endocervix of 3–5% of sexually active women. This provides for additional exposure during the birth process. There is a steady acquisition of CMV from birth to the reproductive age, by which time 50% of women have serologic evidence of prior infection.[8]

Symptoms

CMV is usually asymptomatic in adults with intact host defenses. If symptoms occur, they typically include malaise, fever, headache, and myalgia. Laboratory findings may consist of relative lymphocytosis and thrombocytopenia. Moderate elevation in liver enzymes may also occur. Most infections resolve in 2–6 weeks.

Fetal Transmission

CMV can be transmitted to an infant during pregnancy, ingestion of infected human milk, direct contact with urine, blood and saliva. Congenital transmission of CMV can occur with primary infection, reactivation or recurrent maternal infection during pregnancy, although the risk of congenital infection is much higher with primary infection (30–40% with primary infection versus less than 1% with recurrent infection). The fetus can be affected at any stage of pregnancy, but the effects are most severe when it occurs early.

Fetal Sequelae

10 to 15 per cent of infants with congenital CMV infection are symptomatic at birth.

- *Ocular:* Chorioretinitis, microphthalmia, cataract blindness, optic atrophy.
- *Auditory:* Sensorineural deafness (most common cause of deafness)
- *Hepatic:* Hepatospenomegaly, jaundice
- *Hematological:* Anemia, thrombocytopenia
- *Neurological:* Microcephaly, neuro-developmental delay, cerebral palsy, seizures, learning difficulties.

Diagnosis

Most often, the diagnosis is unsuspected until the birth of an affected infant. Diagnosis is made by paired serological samples by ELSIA or RIA from the mother (Table 24.3).

The gold standard for the diagnosis of congenital CMV infection is a positive amniotic fluid culture. Other tests include detection of the virus from amniotic fluid by PCR, cordocentesis with serological testing for detection of CMV specific IgM in fetal blood.[9]

A diagnosis of fetal CMV infection can be made if the virus is found in the infant's urine, saliva, blood or other body tissues 2–3 weeks after birth.

Treatment

Currently, there is no effective therapy for CMV infection during pregnancy. Treatment with ganciclovir during pregnancy has not been shown to prevent congenital CMV infection.[10] Valcyclovir 1 gm twice daily for 10 days has been used but more data are needed. Women should be thoroughly counseled about the risk of fetal damage and the need to consider invasive procedures to establish the fetal risk. If affected, one should consider termination of pregnancy. Further, serial ultrasound scans should be arranged to detect fetal abnormalities—echogenic bowel, microcephaly, intracranial calcifications and IUGR. However, a normal scan does not guarantee a normal baby and all infected fetuses may not be affected.

Recent studies by Nigro and colleagues have shown a significant reduction in both the incidence and severity of congenital CMV with the use of passive immunization with hyperimmune globulin[11] (CMV HIG). There is no specific therapy for the affected newborn though neonatal treatment with ganciclovir showed prevention of hearing loss progression.

The algorithm for the diagnosis and treatment for CMV infection is shown in Fig. 24.5.

HERPES SIMPLEX VIRUS

The infection is covered in detail in the respective chapter.

Others

Other infections in the TORCH group include parvovirus, varicella zoster virus, hepatitis virus, syphilis.

Varicella zoster virus and hepatitis virus are covered in respective chapters.

Parvovirus

Causative Organism

It is a non-enveloped single-stranded DNA virus that causes erythema infectiosum (fifth disease) in children.

Mode of Infection

Infection is transmitted through air and contaminated blood. Infection of a negative mother occurs due to contact with children

Table 24.3: Diagnosis		
	IgM	*IgG*
Primary infection	Detected by 2 weeks	Detected by 2 weeks
	Persists for 4–9 months	Persists for a lifetime
Recurrent infection	Absence of IgM	Fourfold rise in IgG titres

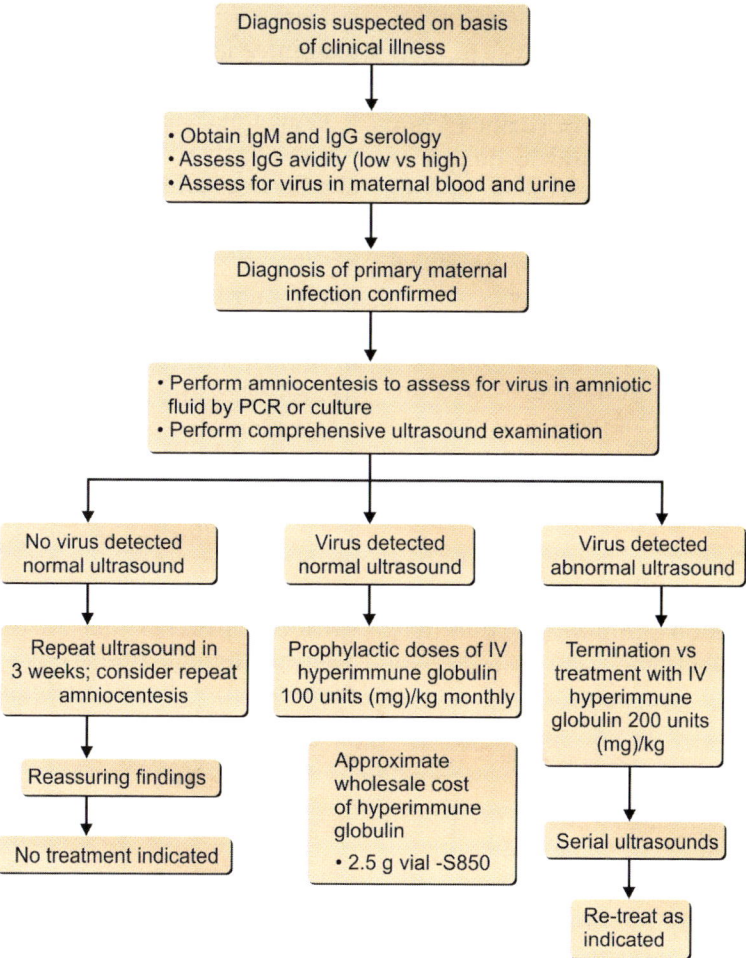

Fig. 24.5: CMV infection

having Erythema infectiosum infection. Incubation period is 4–14 days. The phase of viral replication and shedding occurs prior to the development of symptoms.

Clinical Manifestations

In adults, the presentation may consist of flu-like symptoms including low grade fever, malaise, and headache. Arthralgia may also occur. Approximately 25% of infected adults are asymptomatic. Immunocompromised adults, however, may develop chronic parvovirus B19 infection with anemia and aplastic crisis.

Fetal Transmission and Sequelae

The risk of vertical transmission to the fetus is 33%.[12] Fetal infection may also result in spontaneous abortion and stillbirth.[12] Parvovirus has a predisposition for fetal erythroid progenitor cells inducing cell cycle arrest at the G1 and G2 phases. Damage to red blood cell precursors leads to severe anemia. Severe anemia and tissue hypoxia can lead to high output cardiac failure and fetal hydrops. Myocarditis may be another pathway to fetal cardiac failure. Non-immune hydrops occur in approximately 3% of infected fetuses.

Diagnosis

For routine diagnosis, the serological investigations of amniotic fluid, fetal blood or tissue of the infant are carried out using ELISA and RIA methods. Ultrasound technique is performed to detect the development of fetal hydrops. Amniocentesis, with PCR to detect parvovirus DNA, can be used to diagnose fetal infection.

In the late second and third trimesters, weekly ultrasound examinations to search for evidence of hydrops and to evaluate the middle cerebral artery Doppler evaluation can be used to identify fetal anemia from velocimetry of the middle cerebral artery.[12]

Treatment

There is no specific treatment for B19 virus infection; intravenous immunoglobulin may be beneficial for the same.

SYPHILIS

Causative Organism

It is caused by gram negative spirochete *Treponema pallidum* (*T. pallidum*), 6–15 micron in length.

Mode of Infection

It is spread through direct contact with a spirochete containing lesion, sexually, or transplacentally. Syphilis affects pregnant women in three stages:

- Primary stage—appearance of the syphilitic chancre and lymphadenitis.
- Secondary stage—rash on the hands and feet even after 2–10 weeks of chancre heals.
- Tertiary stage—neurological, cardiovascular, and gummatous lesions (granuloma of the skin and musculoskeletal system).

Fetal Transmission

Congenital syphilis is transmitted from women to the fetus in those having primary and secondary stages of the disease rather than tertiary stage. The determining factor for fetal infection is the degree of spirochetemia in the mother.

Congenital syphilis can be divided into two phases: Early disease (before two years) and late disease (after two years).

Symptoms

Early manifestation include hemorrhagic nasal discharge (sniffles), hepatosplenomegaly, jaundice, lymphadenopathy, hemolytic anemia, thrombocytopenia, osteochondritis and periostitis, mucocutanous rash, CNS abnormalities, failure to thrive, chorioretinitis and nephrotic syndrome.

Late manifestations have signed such as Hutchinson teeth (small teeth with an abnormal central groove), mulberry molars (bulbous protrusions on the molar teeth resembling mulberries), hard palate perforation, eighth nerve deafness, interstitial keratitis, bony lesion, and saber shins (due to chronic periosteitis).

Diagnosis

Diagnosis of syphilis can be performed using dark-field microscopy or using direct immunofluorescence assay of the sample taken from lesions, placenta or umbilicus. Nontreponemal tests are the venereal disease research laboratory (VDRL) and rapid plasma reagin (RPR) tests.

Treponemal tests include the fluorescent treponemal antibody absorption (FTA-ABS) assay and the microhaemagglutination assay for *T. pallidum* antibody (MHA-TP).

Newer methods such as enzyme immunoassay (EIA), PCR, and immunoblott are used; they have greater sensitivity and specificity.

Treatment

In general, treatment of congenital syphilis requires a 10 days course of Penicillin (aqueous penicillin G 100000 to 150000 units/kg/24 hours). Proper treatment of the mother eliminates the risk of infection of infants. The infected infant should be followed up routinely until nontreponemal test reported negative.

Recommendations

- Routine universal screening for toxoplasmosis should not be performed for pregnant women at low risk.

- Suspected recent infection in a pregnant woman should be confirmed before intervention by having samples tested at a toxoplasmosis reference laboratory, using tests that are as accurate as possible and correctly interpreted.

- Rubella susceptibility screening should be offered early in antenatal care to identify women at risk of contracting rubella infection and to enable vaccination in the postnatal period for the protection of future pregnancies.

- Diagnosis of primary maternal cytomegalovirus (CMV) infection in pregnancy should be based on de-novo appearance of virus-specific IgG in the serum of a pregnant woman who was previously seronegative, or on detection of specific IgM antibody associated with low IgG avidity.

- The prenatal diagnosis of fetal CMV infection should be based on amniocentesis, which should be done at least 7 weeks after presumed time of maternal infection and after 21 weeks of gestation. This interval is important because it takes 5 to 7 weeks following fetal infection and subsequent replication of the virus in the kidney for a detectable quantity of the virus to be secreted to the amniotic fluid.

REFERENCES

1. Mccarthy M. Of cats and women. Br Med J (Clin Res Ed) 1983; 287(6390): 445–446.
2. Cook Aj, Gilbert Re, Buffolano W, Zufferey J, Petersen E, Jenum Pa, Foulon W, Semprini Ae, Dunn Dt. Sources of toxoplasma infection in pregnant women: European multicentre case-control study. Br Med J 2000; 321(7254): 142–147.
3. Grover CM, Thulliez P, Remington JS, et al: Rapid prenatal diagnosis of congenital *Toxoplasma* infection by using polymerase chain reaction and amniotic fluid. J Clin Microb 28: 2297, 1990.
4. Puder KS, Treadwell MC, Gonik B: Ultrasound characteristics of in utero infection. Infect Dis Obstet Gynecol 5: 262, 1997.
5. Jean-Benjamin Murat, Hélène Fricker Hidalgo, Marie-Pierre Brenier-Pinchart, Hervé Pelloux Expert Rev Anti Infect Ther. 2013;11(9):943–956.
6. Daffos F, Forestier F, Capella-Pavlovsky M, et al. Prenatal management of 746 pregnancies at risk for congenital toxoplasmosis. N Engl J Med 1988; 31: 271–275.
7. Centers for Disease Control: Rubella vaccination during pregnancy B United States 1971–1988. MMWR Morb Mortal Wkly Rep 38:289, 1989.
8. Cannon MJ, Hyde TB, Schmid DS. Review of cytomegalovirus shedding in bodily fluids and relevance to congenital cytomegalovirus infection. Rev Med Virol. 2011 Jul; 21(4):240–55.
9. Weiner CP, Grose C: Prenatal diagnosis of congenital cytomegalovirus infection by virus isolation from amniotic fluid. Am J Obstet Gynecol 163: 1253, 1990.
10. Revello MG, Gerna G: Diagnosis and implications of human cytomegalovirus infections in pregnancy. Fetal Matern Med Rev 1999; 11: 117–34.
11. Nigro G, Adler SP, La Torre R, Best AM; Congenital Cytomegalovirus Collaborating Group. Passive immunization during pregnancy for congenital cytomegalovirus infection. N Engl J Med. 2005 Sep 29;353(13):1350–62.
12. Cosmi E, Mari G, Chaie LD, et al: Noninvasive diagnosis by Doppler ultrasonography of fetal anemia resulting from parvovirus infection. Am J Obstet Gynecol 2002; 187: 1290–3.

25

Tuberculosis in Pregnancy—Current Guidelines

Vinaya S Karkhanis, Unnati Desai

INTRODUCTION

Tuberculosis (TB) is the leading infectious disease globally and amongst women it still remains an important cause of non-obstetric deaths. Maternal mortality is high among women co-infected with human immuno-deficiency virus (HIV) and TB both during pregnancy and postpartum. India is a high burden country for TB and the estimated annual prevalence and incidence of TB is 211 and 171 per lakh population respectively.[1] Annual rate of TB infection is 1.1% in general population as against 0.1 to 1.9% in pregnant women. The estimated epidemiological prevalence data from India as per World Health Organisation (WHO) 2011 suggests rate of active TB in pregnancy as 2·3 (1·6–3·1) per 1000 pregnant women and 20·6% of global cases burden amongst pregnant women being accounted by India.[1] Delay in diagnosis and inappropriate management of TB in pregnancy is associated with poor outcomes in both mother and the neonate. Obstetric complications of untreated TB include spontaneous abortion, small for date uterus, preterm labour, low birth weight, and increased neonatal mortality. Prompt diagnosis and treatment of TB are essential to prevent maternal and neonatal morbidity and mortality.

IMPACT OF TB ON PREGNANCY

Current medical opinion holds that TB and pregnancy do not affect each other's course, though active TB has adverse obstetrical and neonatal outcomes.[2] Pregnancy in patients with untreated active TB is at high-risk of prematurity, fetal growth retardation, low birth weight and increased perinatal mortality.[3] The pulmonary and extra-pulmonary forms of TB affect the pregnant woman in the same way as in non-pregnant state. The outcome of appropriately treated cases is same as that in non-pregnant patients. Infants born to mothers suffering from TB are at risk of acquiring congenital TB. Prompt diagnosis is essential as half of the neonates delivered with congenital TB may eventually die, especially in the absence of treatment. Congenital tuberculosis is diagnosed by "Cantwell criteria" and treatment includes three or four anti-tubercular drug regimen. In suspected cases morphological, histopatho-logical and microbiological examination of placenta at the time of delivery is helpful in diagnosis. Bacillus Calmette-Guérin (BCG) vaccination is recommended at birth. If there is no active tuberculosis, the infants born to mothers with active TB should receive prophylaxis with isoniazid (H) (5 mg/kg dose) for 3 months or until mother's sputum conversion. After 3 months, if the infant is mantoux test positive, H prophylaxis should be continued for total duration of 6 months after ruling out active tuberculosis.

CLINICAL PRESENTATION OF TB IN PREGNANCY

The clinical profile of TB in pregnancy is similar to that in the general population. The range of symptoms depends on whether it is pulmonary tuberculosis (PTB) or extra pulmonary TB and the site of involvement. A patient presenting with cough for more than 15 days (when other causes of chronic cough are ruled out) is defined as a case of presumptive TB. Definitions in tuberculous disease have been revised in 2013 by the WHO and mentioned in Table 25.1.[4] Cough, fever and hemoptysis are common symptoms of presentation in PTB. In case of extra-pulmonary TB, lymph node is the commonest site involved. Other sites of involvement may present with pleural, spinal, abdominal, central nervous system (CNS) symptoms. Disseminated and miliary TB has multifocal organ involvement with fever, anemia, hepato-megaly and splenomegaly. Non-specific symptoms such as fatigue, altered bowel habits, failure to gain weight may simulate symptoms of pregnancy and can delay diagnosis.

Table 25.1: Definitions in tuberculosis

Definition	Explanation
A bacteriologically confirmed **TB** case	A biological specimen is positive by smear microscopy, culture or WRD
A clinically diagnosed TB case	Not bacteriologically confirmed but diagnosed with active TB by a clinician or other medical practitioner who has decided to give the patient a full course of TB treatment
Pulmonary tuberculosis	Any TB case with involvement of the lung parenchyma or the tracheobronchial tree. Includes miliary and mixed PTB/eartrapulmonary
Extrapulmonary tuberculosis	Any **TB** case with involvement of organs other than the lungs, e.g. pleura, lymph nodes, abdomen, genitourinary tract, skin, joints and bones, meninges
New	Never been treated for TB or have taken anti-TB drugs for less than 1 month
Previously treated	Have received 1 month or more of anti-TB drugs in the past
Relapse	Previously treated for TB, were declared ***cured*** or ***treatment completed*** at the end of their most recent course of treatment, and now diagnosed with a recurrent episode of TB (either a true relapse or a new episode of TB caused by reinfection)
Treatment after failure	Previously treated for TB and whose ***treatment failed*** at the ***end*** of the most recent course of treatment
Treatment after loss to follow-up	Previously treated for TB and ***lost to follow-up*** at the ***end*** of the most recent course of treatment
Other previously treated	Previously treated for TB but whose outcome after the most recent course of treatment is unknown or undocumented
Rifampicin resistance	Resistance to rifampicin detected using phenotypic or genotypic methods, with or without resistance to other anti-TB drugs
Multidrug resistance	Resistance to at least both isoniazid and rifampicin
Extensive drug resistance	Resistance to any fluoroquinolone **and** to at least one of three second-line injectable drugs (capreomycin, kanamycin and amikacin), in addition to multidrug resistance
Monoresistance	Resistance to one first-line anti-TB drug only other than Rifampicin
Polydrug resistance	Resistance to more than one first-line anti-TB drug (other than both isoniazid and rifampicin)

WRD—WHO recognized rapid diagnostics

The diagnosis of TB historically relies on the identification of AFB through microscopic examination of stained sputum smears. The diagnostic algorithm for diagnosis of PTB is illustrated in Fig. 25.1. Smears may be prepared directly from clinical specimens or from concentrated preparations. Two staining methods can be used to observe AFB: Ziehl-Neelsen (ZN) staining or fluorescent auramine staining. However, sputum microscopy has its own limitations. While it is highly specific, sensitivity depends on the quality of sputum sample submitted. Explaining the patients to submit two deeply coughed out or induced (after hypertonic saline nebulisation) mucoid sputum samples (early morning and spot) with at least 5 ml quantity improves the sensitivity. 24-hour sputum may be collected in patients not able to produce satisfactory sputum. Induction of sputum with hypertonic saline nebulisation yields favourable results to avoid unnecessary bronchoscopies.[5] Improper sputum collection, i.e. saliva sent for examination adds to the burden on laboratories and unnecessary delay in diagnosis. WHO recognised rapid diagnostics (WRD) such as molecular deoxyribonucleic acid (DNA) detection methods like GeneXpert (GXP) may be used as an add-on test to microscopy, especially in smear-negative specimens (conditional recommendation, recognising major resource implications). For patients suspected of having extrapulmonary TB, specimens should be obtained from the suspected sites either by fine needle aspiration cytology (FNAC) or fine needle aspiration biopsy (FNAB), excision biopsy or surgery, for histopathological and microbiological examination for GXP and AFB culture. Chest X-ray may be done only in complicated cases with appropriate precautions in view of radiation exposure. In settings where WRDs like GXP and line probe assay (LPA) are available, MDR-TB should be essentially confirmed or excluded within 1–2 days and the results should guide treatment regimen at start of therapy. Modification of the diagnostic algorithm integrating GXP (where facility is available) in the evaluation is illustrated in Fig. 25.2. Multi-drug resistant TB (MDR-TB) can be diagnosed by GXP testing with simultaneous smear or liquid culture line probe assay (LPA) for drug susceptibility study (DST) of INH (H), Rifampicin (R),

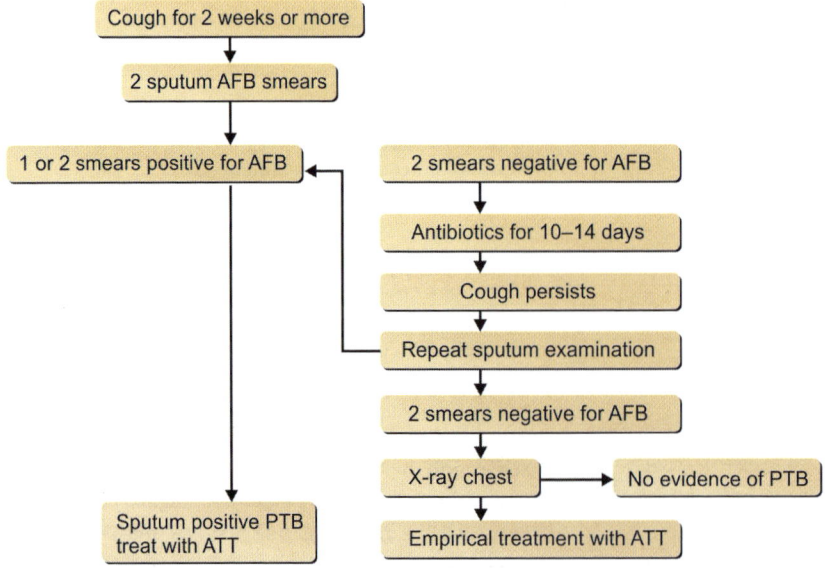

Fig. 25.1: Diagnostic algorithm for diagnosis of PTB

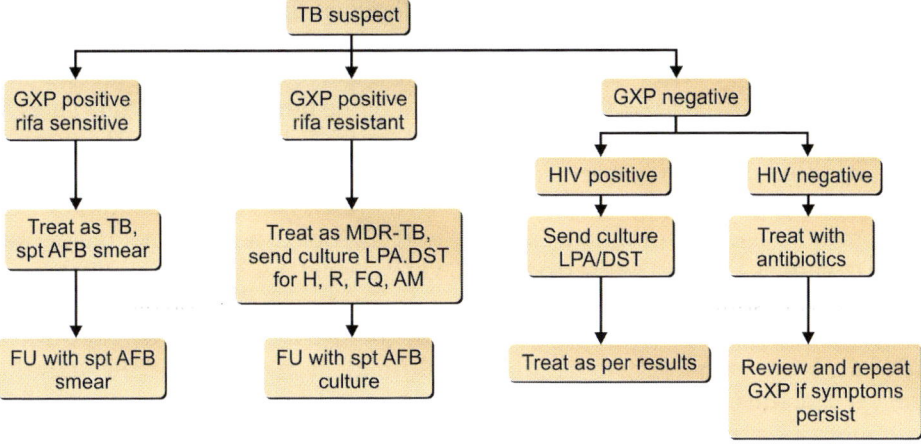

Fig. 25.2: Modification of diagnostic algorithm integrating GXP

Kanamycin (Km), and Ofloxacin (Ofx) from accredited laboratories. DST results for other second line drugs are not reliable. Mantoux test (MT) is not diagnostic of active TB but can be used as surrogate evidence in sympto-matics with extra pulmonary involvement and in HIV positive patients for diagnosing latent TB infection. Interferon-gamma release assays (IGRAs), another diagnostic tool for diagnosis of latent infection, are in vitro blood tests. IGRAs cannot distinguish between latent infection and active TB disease and should not replace the standard diagnostic methods including microbiology, molecular tests for diagnosis of active TB.[6] WHO states that blood-based antibody tests like IgG/IgM enzyme linked immunosorbent assay (ELISA) and IGRAs like TB-GOLD are not accurate and should not be used for TB diagnosis.[7]

TREATMENT OF TB DURING PREGNANCY

Treatment regimen and duration therapy of pulmonary and extrapulmonary TB is same as in general population, including in HIV positive patients on anti-retroviral therapy (ART). "Untreated tuberculosis represents a far greater hazard to a pregnant woman and her fetus than does treatment of the disease".[8] Compliance with therapy is essential for successful treatment of TB. Prior counseling regarding disease status, therapy duration and related adverse effects ensures compliance. All drugs need to be taken together to achieve peak therapeutic concentration of the drugs. The short course chemotherapy (SCC) comprising drugs like R, H, ethambutol (E), and pyrazinamide (Z) can be used safely during pregnancy. Streptomycin (SM) is not given as it can cause ototoxicity to the fetus. Addition of pyridoxine in the dose of 10 mg/day is recommended to prevent H related peripheral neuropathy. The treatment of TB depends on the previous history of anti-tuberculosis treatment (ATT). The WHO guidelines[7] state: New pregnant patients with tuberculosis should receive a regimen containing 6 months of R: 2HRZE/4HR (Strong/High grade of evidence). This 6 months regimen containing 4 drugs for 2 months of intensive phase (IP) followed by 2 drugs for 4 months continuation phase (CP) is also known as SCC. Alternately if daily therapy needs to be given fixed dose combinations (FDCs) are a preferable option as they prevent acquisition of drug resistance due to monotherapy which may occur with separate "loose" drugs. FDCs reduce prescription errors and decrease pill burden to improve patient adherence to therapy. Recommended doses of first-line anti-TB drugs for pregnant women are given in

Table 25.2. In previously treated patients, after MDR-TB is ruled out retreatment regimen containing 3HRZE/5HRE should be prescribed. If diagnosed as MDR-TB on DST, regimens should be adjusted appropriately. Regimens are illustrated in Table 25.3. To assess treatment response, the WHO guidelines[7] recommend: For pregnant smear-positive PTB patients treated with first-line drugs, sputum smear microscopy may be performed at completion IP of treatment (Conditional/high or moderate grade of evidence), i.e. 2 months in new cases, 3 months in retreatment cases. If results are negative further sputum smear microscopy is recommended at the end of therapy. In new patients, if the specimen obtained at the end of the IP (month 2) is smear-positive, sputum smear microscopy should be obtained at the end of the third month (strong/high grade of evidence)." At the end of IP either in new or retreatment cases if sputum remains positive, WRD tests (GXP, LPA) should be performed and referral to a pulmonologist is advisable. GXP should not be used in follow up cases to interpret microbiological conversion. For pregnant patients with extrapulmonary TB, clinical monitoring is the usual way of assessing the response to treatment as radiological imaging has its limitations. Treatment outcomes are listed in Table 25.4. Common adverse drug reactions to ATT are

Table 25.2: Recommended doses of first-line and second-line antituberculosis drugs for pregnant women

Drug		Recommended dose		
		Daily		Thrice weekly
	Dose and range (mg/kg body weight)	Maximum (mg)	Dose and range (mg/kg body weight)	Maximum (mg)
Rifampicin	10 (8–12)	600	10 (8–12)	600
Isoniazid	5 (4–6)	300	10 (8–12)	900
Ethambutol	15 (15–20)	–	30 (25–35)	–
Pyrazinamide	25 (20–30)	–	35 (30–40)	–
Fluoroquinolones	15	1000		
Ethionamide	15	1000	Not applicable	
Cycloserine	15	1000		
Paraaminosalicylic acid (PAS)	150 of elemental PAS	16 gm		

Streptomycin and kanamycin are contraindicated in pregnancy, ethionamide is contraindicated in first trimester

Table 25.3: Regimens for treatment of tuberculosis for pregnant patients

Regimen	Duration (months)	Regimen
New patient	2 IP, 4 CP	2 HRZE/4 HR
Retreatment with first-line drugs	3 IP, 5 CP	3 HRZE/5 HRE
MDR TB	6–9 IP, 18 CP	Cyc *Eto Levo PAS E Z/Cyc, Eto, Levo, PAS
XDRTB	6–12 IP, 18 CP	PAS, Mfx, high dose INH, Cfz, Lzd, Amx-clv/ PAS, Mfx, high dose INH, Cfz, Lzd, Amx-clv

IP-Intensive phase, CP-Continuation phase

H-Isoniazid, R-rifampicin, Z-pyrazinamide, E-ethambutol, Cyc-cycloserine, Eto-ethionamide, Levo-levofloxacin, PAS-para-amino salicylic acid, moxifloxacin (Mfx), clofazimine(Cfz), linezolid (Lzd) and amoxyclav (Amx/clv)

Streptomycin and kanamycin are contraindicated in pregnancy

*Ethionamide is contraindicated in the first trimester

listed in Table 25.5. Special situations of hepatitis, renal derangement and serious cutaneous reactions in pregnant patients of TB warrant a specialist referral for therapy modification. Steroids may be indicated in conditions like adrenal insufficiency, pericardial effusions, idiosyncratic reactions, CNS tuberculosis, and severe forms of miliary TB especially with paradoxical responses. Steroid dose needs to be doubled when given with "R," taking drug interactions in consideration. Paradoxical reactions while on therapy with worsening of the pre-existing disease; clinically or radiologically add to suspicion of MDR-TB. These are due to significant reduction of mycobacterial load after initiation of ATT due to release of large amount of tuberculoproteins and other cell wall products. This causes a cellular and cytokine inflammatory response, leading to local tissue damage and paradoxical phenomenon.[9] Patient needs to be reassured and same therapy is continued. "Addition and deletion phenomenon", i.e. addition or deletion of single drug to failing regimen should be strictly avoided as it adds to emergence of drug resistance. MDR-TB may be excluded with WRD like GXP and smear or culture LPA-DST. Pleural, lymph node and CNS involvement are very common.[9] They are usually self limiting and does not warrant change in therapy. But sometimes if

Table 25.4: Definition of treatment outcomes	
Outcome	Definition
Cure	A patient whose sputum smear or culture was positive at the beginning of the treatment but who was smear- or culture-negative in the last month of treatment **and** on at least one previous occasion
Treatment completed	A patient who completed treatment but who does not have a negative sputum smear or culture result in the last month of treatment and on at least one previous occasion
Treatment failure	A patient whose sputum smear or culture is positive at 5 months or later during treatment. Also included in this definition are patients found to harbour a multidrug-resistant **(MDR)** strain at **any** point of time during the treatment, whether they are smear-negative or -positive
Died	A patient who dies for any reason during the course of treatment
Default	A patient whose treatment was interrupted for 2 consecutive months or more
Transfer out	A patient who has been transferred to another recording and reporting unit and whose treatment outcome is unknown
Treatment success	A sum of cured and completed treatment

Table 25.5: Common adverse drug reactions to first-line and second-line ATT	
Drug	Adverse drug reactions
Rifampicin	Hepatotoxicity, gastrointestinal, autoimmune reactions like flu syndrome, thrombocytopenia, purpura, respiratory syndrome, acute hemolytic anemia, acute renal failure
Isoniazid	Hepatotoxicity, peripheral neuritis, hypersensitive reactions may precipitate epilepsy, drug induced lupus, psychotic changes
Ethambutol	Optic neuritis, color blindness, gastrointestinal, allergic reactions, hyperuricemia
Pyrazinamide	Hepatotoxicity, arthralgia, hyperuricemia, gastrointestinal, allergic reactions
Fluoroquinolones	GI upset, dizziness, hypersensitivity, drug interactions, headaches, restlessness
Ethionamide	GI upset, hepatotoxicity, hypersensitivity, metallic taste
Cycloserine	Psychosis, convulsions, depression, headaches, rash, drug interactions
PAS	GI upset, hypersensitivity, hepatotoxicity, sodium load

unrecognized, can lead to mortality; especially in cases of miliary and CNS TB where treatment with steroids is indicated.

DRUG RESISTANT TUBERCULOSIS

"R" resistance or MDR-TB are synonymous as both are associated with failure of SCC. Over 90% of "R" resistance is linked to "H" resistance, and the number is even higher in patients who have already been treated. On the contrary "H" resistance is linked to "R" resistance in a small percentage of patients. Patients with "H" monoresistance can be treated successfully with standard SCC.[10] MDR-TB is diagnosed when organisms show resistance to at least H and R. Term XDR-TB (extensive drug resistance) is used when there is resistance to one of the injectable aminoglycosides and fluoroquinolone in addition to H and R resistance. The prevalence of primary MDR is 2–3% and acquired MDR is 12–17%. Primary resistance in TB refers to patients infected with mycobacterium tuberculosis that is resistant to anti-TB drugs from the outset, prior to anti-TB treatment. The emergence of acquired resistance involves selective mutation of an organism due to inappropriate regimens, use of lower than recommended dosage, poor drug quality and poor adherence to treatment. MDR-TB is suspected when a case of TB is smear/culture positive for AFB in spite of adequate duration of first-line ATT; suggesting treatment failure or when there is a contact with a case of proven MDR-TB. Diagnosis of MDR-TB can be done with the help of WHO recommended DST which include rapid diagnostic tests like GXP, smear LPA, liquid culture LPA or solid culture. The diagnostic test algorithm for MDR-TB is summarized in Table 25.6. WHO recommends universal access of DST for all patients of TB; however, logistic and programmatic implementations of DST referral for MDR suspects depend on the resources available in the area. Once diagnosed as MDR, patients are referred to the Drug Resistant Tuberculosis (DR-TB) centers for pretreatment evaluation (i.e. complete blood count, HIV, blood sugar, thyroid function test, renal function tests, liver function tests, urine examination for routine microscopy and urinary pregnancy test), and initiation of category IV (second-line anti-tuberculous therapy). There is paucity of data on the efficacy and safety of second-line drugs during pregnancy, and the management of

Test	Time for diagnosis	Principle
GeneXpert (GXP)	90 minutes	Cartridge based automated nucleic acid amplification test. Sensitivity- 98%, specificity-98%
Line probe assay (LPA) DST	48–72 hours	PCR hybridization technique which identifies drug-resistant strains by detecting the most common single nucleotide polymorphisms (SNPs) associated with resistance. Sensitivity-99%, specificity-97%
Liquid culture (MGIT) and LPA DST	20–45 days	Replaced the solid AFB culture & DST for diagnosis. BACTEC- 460 radiometric method, mycobacterial growth indicator tube (MGIT- 960 system)
Solid AFB culture and LPA DST	45–70 days	Gold standard. Now used mainly for research purpose. Various methods like proportion, absolute concentration, resistance ratio
Liquid culture and liquid DST	45–70 days	
Solid culture (LJ medium) and DST	84 days	

Table 25.6: Preference of diagnostic tests for drug resistance

DST- Drug susceptibility tests, MGIT- Mycobacteria growth indicator tube, LJ-medium- Lowenstein-Jensen medium

MDR-TB during pregnancy remains controversial. Second-line TB drugs used to treat MDR-TB, such as aminoglycosides, are ototoxic and nephrotoxic for both the mother and the fetus. Quinolones have teratogenic potential and cause skeletal deformities. There are no safety data from human studies for the new TB drugs bedaquiline and delamanid, limiting their usefulness in treating pregnant women with MDR-TB.[11] The algorithm is guided by WHO and RNTCP's Programmatic management of TB (PMDT) guidelines.[12] Management decisions for MDR-TB patients who are pregnant prior to initiation of treatment or whilst on treatment are based on the duration of pregnancy. If the duration of pregnancy is <20 weeks, the patient should be advised to opt for a Medical Termination of Pregnancy (MTP) in view of the potential severe risk to both the mother and fetus. If the patient is willing, she should be referred to a Gynaecologist/Obstetrician for MTP following which treatment can be initiated (if the patient has not started treatment) or continued (if the patient is already on treatment). For patients who are unwilling for MTP or have pregnancy of >20 weeks (making them ineligible for MTP), the risk to the mother and fetus needs to be explained clearly and a modified regimen for MDR-TB is prescribed. The standard regimen for MDR-TB, category IV, consists of 6–9 months of IP consisting of kanamycin (Km), levofloxacin (Lvx), ethionamide (Eto), cycloserine (Cs), ethambutol (E), pyrazinamide (Z) followed by 18 months of CP consisting of Lvx, Eto, Cs and E. For pregnant patients in the first trimester (less than 12 weeks), Km and Eto are omitted from the regimen and Para-aminosalicylic acid (PAS) is added. For patients who have completed the first trimester (>12 weeks), only Km is replaced with PAS. Postpartum, PAS may be replaced with Km and continued until the end of IP. Flow chart for management of MDR-TB during pregnancy is illustrated in Fig. 25.3. XDR-TB patients should undergo pre-treatment evaluation identical to MDR-TB patients with addition of ECG, serum electrolyte testing. The regimen constitute 6–12 months of intensive phase with PAS, moxifloxacin (Mfx), high dose H, clofazimine (Cfz), linezolid (Lzd) and amoxyclav (Amx/clv) and 18 months of continuation phase with PAS, Mfx, high dose H, Cfz, Lzd and Amx/clv. Change from IP to CP is done only after achievement of culture conversion, with 2 consecutive negative cultures at least one

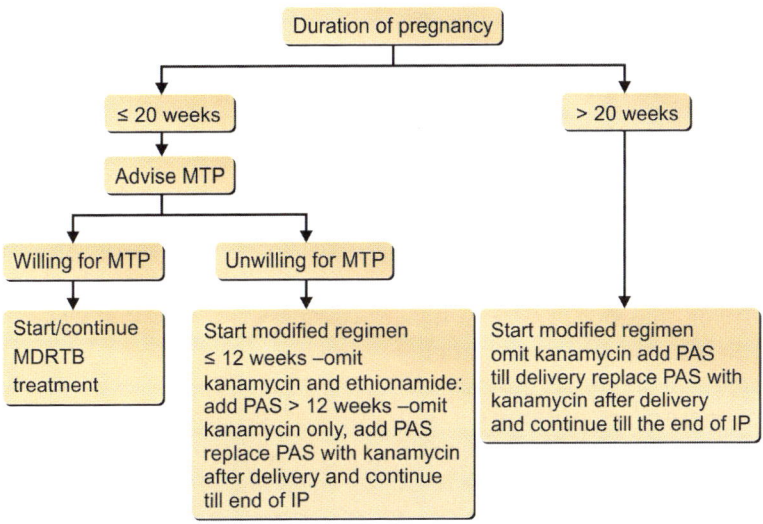

Fig. 25.3: Management of MDR-TB during pregnancy

month apart. Dosages of second-line ATT are given in Table 25.2. Common adverse drug reactions to second-line ATT are enumerated in Table 25.5. Patients need hospitalization in case of severe adverse reactions to drugs. Pregnant MDR-TB patients need to be monitored carefully both in relation to the treatment and the progress of the pregnancy. If the patient is sputum smear-negative at the time of parturition, mother and infant need not to be separated and breastfeeding should be encouraged. However, if the patient is sputum smear-positive at parturition, barrier nursing should be advised to prevent transmission of infection. The American Academy of Pediatrics (AAP) recommends that women with tuberculosis who have been treated appropriately for two weeks or more and who are not considered contagious may breastfeed,[13] while the WHO recommends breast-feeding of neonates regardless of the mother's TB status, however, close contact with the baby should be reduced.[7]

PREGNANCY WITH HIV-TB CO-INFECTION

The effects of tuberculosis among pregnant women living with HIV include a 2.2–3.2-fold and 3.4-fold increase in maternal and infant mortality, respectively, compared with HIV-negative women. In addition it adds to the 2.5 fold risk of vertical transmission of HIV. Over 50% of the maternal mortality occurring in mothers with TB in pregnancy is due to co-infection with HIV. The diagnosis of TB in HIV infected pregnant women follows the same diagnostic algorithm as in an HIV non-infected; however, the use of WRD and AFB cultures is recommended in all suspected TB patients with HIV co-infection. The treatment guidelines for co-infected pregnant patients are generalised from those recommended universally for general population. Drug Interaction between R and non-nucleoside reverse transcriptase inhibitors (NNRTIs) and protease inhibitors (PIs) may cause a reduction in the serum concentration leading to ART failure. Nevirapine (NVP) regimen need to be switched over to Efavirenz (EFV) because of "R"-containing ATT and shifted back to NVP after completion of the TB treatment.[14] MDR-TB-HIV co-infection patients need prompt diagnosis and commencement of ATT, co-trimoxazole preventive therapy, and referral for ART. ART should be started as soon as TB treatment is tolerated, within 8 weeks of anti-tuberculosis treatment to avoid related mortality. Paradoxical reactions following the initiation of highly active antiretroviral therapy (HAART), described as "immune reconstitution inflammatory syndrome" (IRIS) are common with ATT.[15] Asymptomatic patients with MT test positivity (MT >5 mm), need to be treated with H chemoprophylaxis (5 mg/kg) for 6 months duration for latent tuberculosis infection.

REFERENCES

1. Global tuberculosis report 2014. Downloaded from: http://www.who.int/tb/publications/global_report/en/

2. Ormerod P. Tuberculosis in pregnancy and the puerperium. Thorax, 2001; 56:494–9.

3. Jana N, Vasishta K, Jindal SK, Khunnu B, Ghosh K. Perinatal outcome in pregnancies complicated by pulmonary tuberculosis. Int J Gynaecol Obstet, 1994;44(2):119–24.

4. Definitions and reporting framework for tuberculosis.2013 revision. downloaded from www.who.int/iris/bitstream /10665/79199/1 / 978924150534 _eng.pdf

5. SR Olsen, R Long, GJ Tyrrell, D Kunimoto. Induced sputum for the diagnosis of pulmonary tuberculosis: Is it useful in clinical practice? Can Respir J 2010;17(4):e81–e84.

6. Lange C, Pai M, Drobniewski F, Migliori GB. Interferon-gamma release assays in the diagnosis of active tuberculosis: sensible or silly? Eur Respir J 2009; 33:1250–3.

7. World Health Organization. Global tuberculosis control: WHO report 2012. Geneva WHO;2012, report No:9789241564502.

8. Centre for Disease Control, "Treatment of tuberculosis," MMWR 2003; 52, 1–77.

9. Cheng VC, Yam WC, Woo PC, Lau SK, Hung IF, Wong SP, et al. Risk factors for development of paradoxical response during antituberculosis therapy in HIV-negative patients. Eur J Clin Microbiol Infect Dis 2003; 22:597–602.

10. Guidelines for Clinical and Operational Management of Drug-Resistant Tuberculosis, 2013. Downloaded from: http://www.theunion. org/what-we-do/publications /technical/ english/mdr-tbguide_6-19-13_web.pdf

11. Bates M, Ahmed Y, Kapata N, Maeurer M, Mwaba P, Zumla A. Perspectives on tuberculosis in pregnancy. Int J Infect Dis 2015; 32:124–7.

12. Revised National Tuberculosis Programme. Guideline on Programmatic Management of drug resistant tuberculosis (PMDT) in India. Update May 2012 downloaded from http:// www. tbcindia.nic.in/documents.html

13. American Academy of Pediatrics. Tuberculosis. In: Pickering LK, editor. Red book: 2012 report of the committee on infectious diseases. 29th ed. Elk Grove Village, IL: American Academy of Pediatrics; 2012. p. 736–56

14. Antiretroviral therapy guidelines for HIV infected adults and adolescents, NACO 2013. http://www.naco.gov.in

15. Lipman M, Breen R. Immune reconstitution inflammatory syndrome in HIV. Curr Opin Infect Dis 2006; 19: 20–25.

26

Varicella and Pregnancy

Preeta R Yadav

INTRODUCTION

Varicella is one of several infections that has significant consequence for the pregnant woman and her developing fetus.

Exposure of non-immune individuals to Varicella Zoster Virus (VZV) in neonatal and maternity settings can cause serious illness in these relatively compromised high-risk patients.

INCIDENCE

It is a unique herpes virus, a double stranded DNA virus, belonging to subfamily Alphaherpesvirinae. Primarily it is a disease of childhood where 90% cases occur in children younger than 10 years of age and touched with 95% of parturient woman in New York and 95% of HIV-positive men.

A study of pregnant patients with negative or indeterminate history of varicella-like illness demonstrated that 81% will show serologic evidence of subclinical infection. There is a 0.05–0.07% risk in women who reach their child-bearing age without developing immunity to varicella of developing chicken- pox during pregnancy. Incidence of varicella in pregnancy is calculated to be 2–3/1000 pregnancies.

PATHOGENESIS

Varicella virus is highly infectious agent and spread by respiratory droplets as well as direct contact with fluid in vesicles, which is a hallmark of infection. Then it infects the conjunctiva and the mucosa in the upper respiratory tract. This is followed by the first cycle of replication, which takes place in the regional lymph nodes on day 2 through 4, and a primary viremia which occur between day 4 and 6. Next, a second replication cycles follows, which occurs in the liver, spleen and the other organs. Finally, the second viremia occurs which seeds the body with viral particles, the capillary endothelial cells and ultimately the epidermis on approximately days 14 and 16.

CLINICAL FEATURES

The incubation period is 14–16 days (range 10–21 days) from exposure to onset of symptoms. Varicella has got typical skin eruption. It starts with red papules on erythematous base, that progress to become vesicles, looking like, "dew drops on rose petals". Vesicles become cloudy pustules and subsequently dry to form crusted lesions (Fig. 26.1). They are intensely pruritic and occur in crops. The lesions are centripetally distributed, starting from face, trunk and then the extremities. It can precede with prodrome in adult like headache, myalgia, nausea, anorexia and vomiting.

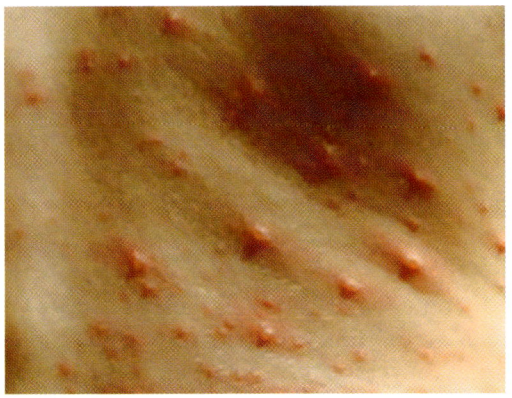

Fig, 26.1: Classical features of varicella in neonates

CLINICAL MANIFESTATIONS

There are two types of pregnant woman:

- One who has previous history of chicken-pox infection, is 97–99% predictive of the presence of serum varicella antibodies, and
- The other who have never had varicella infection in the past and/or have not received varicella vaccine, or in whom varicella antibody is negative. They are non-immune patients. Their management is different.

MATERNAL COMPLICATIONS

During and after mid-pregnancy there is greatest risk of severe illness like pneumonia, hepatitis and encephalitis.

Pneumonia can occur in up to 10–20% of pregnant woman with chickenpox. It is the most common complication. In later gestation the complications increases with mortality rate of 14%, but <1% of adult develop encephalitis.

The factors that increase the risks are immune suppression or more than 100 skin lesions or hemorrhagic lesions. Other factors are: Cigarette smoking, chronic obstructive lung disease, history of taking steroids in preceding 3 months.

Women who develop varicella during pregnancy may experience spontaneous abortion, fetal demise, and congenital anomalies.

Fetal ultrasound scan 5 weeks after primary infection is recommended to all pregnant women who develop varicella during first and second trimester to screen for fetal abnormalities.

Chorionic villus sampling, amniocentesis and cordocentesis do not play an important role in the diagnosis of congenital varicella infection.

FETAL COMPLICATION

First and Second Trimesters

"Fetal varicella syndrome" develops in < 2% of the babies born to mother between 7 and 28 weeks of pregnancy. It has a mortality rate of 30% in the first month of life. It does not occur at the time of initial fetal infections but results from a subsequent herpes zoster reactivation in utero, and only occurs in minority of the infected fetus.

Third Trimester

When maternal infection occurs in the last 3 weeks to more than 5 days before delivery, there is a significant risk (23%) of neonatal varicella despite high titers of passively acquired maternal antibody. The route of infection is transplacental (in first 10–12 days of life); ascending vaginal or direct contact with lesions during or after delivery. There can be infantile shingles in the first few years of life due to activation of virus after primary infection in utero.

Clinically the newborn presents with low birth weight, cutaneous scars in dermatomal patterns, papular lesions, ocular abnormalities, bone and muscle hypoplasia, neurological abnormalities.

Severe varicella at any stage of pregnancy can lead to intrauterine death.

Diagnosis

It is usually made clinically, but viral cultures, direct fluorescent antibodies or Tzanck smears are performed. Nowadays it is confirmed by varicella-zoster serology.

Acute infection—IgM antibody positive, IgG antibody negative.

TREATMENT AND MANAGEMENT
Maternal

Symptomatic treatment is advised in the formed of calamine lotion, tepid baths, cool compresses, and antipyretic (excluding aspirin secondary to association with Reye's syndrome).

Prevention of Varicella in Pregnant Women

- Varicella zoster immunoglobulin (VZIG) which is disease specific immunoglobulin is recommended as post-exposure prophy- laxis for non-immune pregnant women.
- It should be administered within 72–96 hours after exposure to lower varicella infection rates. Protection is estimated to extend through 3 weeks. VZIG has no therapeutic benefit once chickenpox has already developed. Acyclovir, can also be given on the 7th post-exposure day as a preventive therapy, but the prophylactic role of this drug in chickenpox is yet to be established. Oral acyclovir 800 mg orally 5 times daily for 7 days or valacyclovir 1000 mg orally 3 times daily for 7 days. It reduces the maximum number of lesions by 46%.

Varicella vaccine (varivax) is a live attenuated vaccine derived from Oka strain. It is contraindicated in pregnant women or those expected to be pregnant in the next one month. But, termination of pregnancy should not be recommended in case of inadvertent vaccination during pregnancy. Varicella vaccination pre-pregnancy (at least one month prior to conception) or postpartum can be considered for women who are found to be seronegative. (For VZV IgG before pregnancy or in postpartum period refer to Table 26.1.)

TREATMENT OF CHICKENPOX DURING PREGNANCY
Varicella Before 20 Weeks of Pregnancy

Within 24–72 hours of onset of rash, oral acyclovir 800 mg five times a day for 7 days should be started. It is a pregnancy category B drug. It should be used when potential benefits outweigh risk.

If complications of varicella progresses or severity of infection warrants, then intra- venous acyclovir 10–15 mg/kg every 8 hours for 5–10 days can be considered.

After 20 weeks also similar regime of acyclovir is followed.

Date of delivery may be postponed to allow maternal antibodies to pass the placental barrier.

In immunocompromised adult, although vidarabine and parenteral human interferon alfa have been proven to be efficacious. Moreover, its safety is not studied in pregnancy. Significant toxicity have limited their use or not used in pregnancy (neuro- toxicity with vidarabine and fever, myalgia with interferon alpha). No controlled study has yet established the effectiveness of acyclovir or valacyclovir for post-exposure to neonate or pregnant women.

Fetal/Neonatal Varicella

Congenital varicella syndrome: No treatment is effective and there is 30% mortality rate.

Neonatal varicella: Intravenous acyclovir 10–15 mg/kg every 8 hours for 5–7 days to be given within 24 hrs of the onset of rash.

If the newborn has contracted "neonatal varicella", i.e. onset of varicella in mother is 5 days before delivery to 2 days after delivery, an estimated 20–50% of the newborn contract "neonatal varicella" and 30% develop severe neonatal varicella (Fig. 26.2). It does not have enough time to acquire passively transferred maternal antibody. In that case, the neonate should be given prophylactic VZIG imme- diately after birth. With the use of VZIG, the

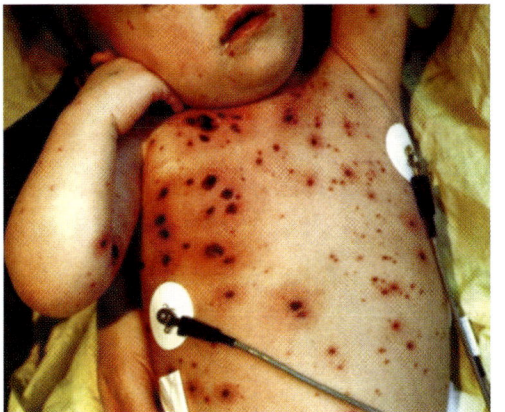

Fig. 26.2: Neonatal varicella

mortality rate has declined from 31% to 7% among neonates with severe varicella infection.

CONCLUSIONS

Varicella is common viral illness in the community, with a significant impact on non-immune pregnant women and their babies.

Therefore, if the patient is uncertain about immunity to varicella, varicella–zoster IgG assay is performed. If IgG is positive, she is reassured that she is immune. If IgG is negative, then she should be offered

Table 26.1: VZIG
VZIG
It is a disease specific immunoglobulin prepared by pooling plasma of donors with high levels of varicella zoster antibody. Each vial of 5 ml contains 125 IU of Immunoglobulin.
It is administered intramuscular as a single dose and a second dose repeated if exposure occurs after 3 weeks.
It is given as post-exposure prophylaxis with a dose of 125 IU/ 10 kg up to maximum dose 625 IU and minimum of 125 IU, in
a. Immunocompromised.
b. Non-immune pregnant women.
c. Neonates whose mother had varicella between 5 days antepartum to 2 days postpartum.
d. Premature infants born at < 28 weeks weighing < 1000 gm at birth and exposed during the neonatal period, irrespective of maternal immunity.
e. Premature infants born at > 28 weeks of gestation who were exposed during the neonatal period and whose mother are non-immune.

Table 26.2: Varicella vaccine
Varicella vaccine
It is a live attenuated varicella virus, prepared from Oka/ Merck strain.
Each vial of 0.5 ml contains 1350–2000 plaque forming units.
It is given as subcutaneous injection.
In Children: 1–< 13 years of age—1 dose, 0.5 ml at 12–15 months, and 2nd dose at 4–6 years of age.
It can also be given with combination with MMR, i.e. MMRV.
Children aged 13 years and Adults—2 doses 4–8 weeks apart.
Women with reproductive age who are susceptible to varicella should be offered the varicella vaccine at the time of their annual examination or preconception counseling appointment. Similarly, susceptible pregnant women should be offered the vaccine immediately after delivery. Contraception is indicated for a minimum of one month after the second dose is administered. Side-effects like fever, inflammation and pain at the site of injection may occur.
Contraindications
• Pregnancy.
• Immunodeficiency disorder (Relative C/I).
• High dose steroid therapy.
• Allergy to neomycin.
• Untreated active tuberculosis.
• Severe systemic illness.

prophylaxis with either VZIG or acyclovir. If she develops infection despite prophylaxis, she should be treated with therapeutic doses of acyclovir for seven days. If serious sequelae develop, then hospitalization done and intravenous acyclovir started. Following treatment serial ultrasound examination should be performed to assess for finding suggestive of congenital varicella.

BIBLIOGRAPHY

1. Pregnancy and Varicella Infection: A resident's quest. Sangita Ghosh, Soumik Choudhary. IJDVL. 2013; Vol. 79/Issue 2/Pg:264–267.
2. CDC; Updated Recommendations for use of VariZIGUnitedstates, 2013.
3. Management of Varicella Infection (Chickenpox) in Pregnancy. Alon Shrim, MD, Gideon Koren, et al. J Obstet Gynaecol Can. 2012; 34(3); 287–292.
4. Varicella Zoster Virus (Chickenpox) Infection in Pregnancy. Ronald F. Laumont, Jack D. Sobel, D Carrington et al. BJOG. 2011 Sept;118(10): 1155–1162.
5. Diagnosis and Management of Varicella Infection in Pregnancy. Patrick Duff, MD, Perinatology 2010; 1:6–12.
6. Varicella and the pregnant women: Prevention and management. Andrew Daley, Thorpe S, Garland SM, Australian NZJ, Obstet Gynaecol 2008 Feb; 48(1): 26–33.

Appendix: Initial rapid diagnosis, assessment and treatment of malaria in pregnancy

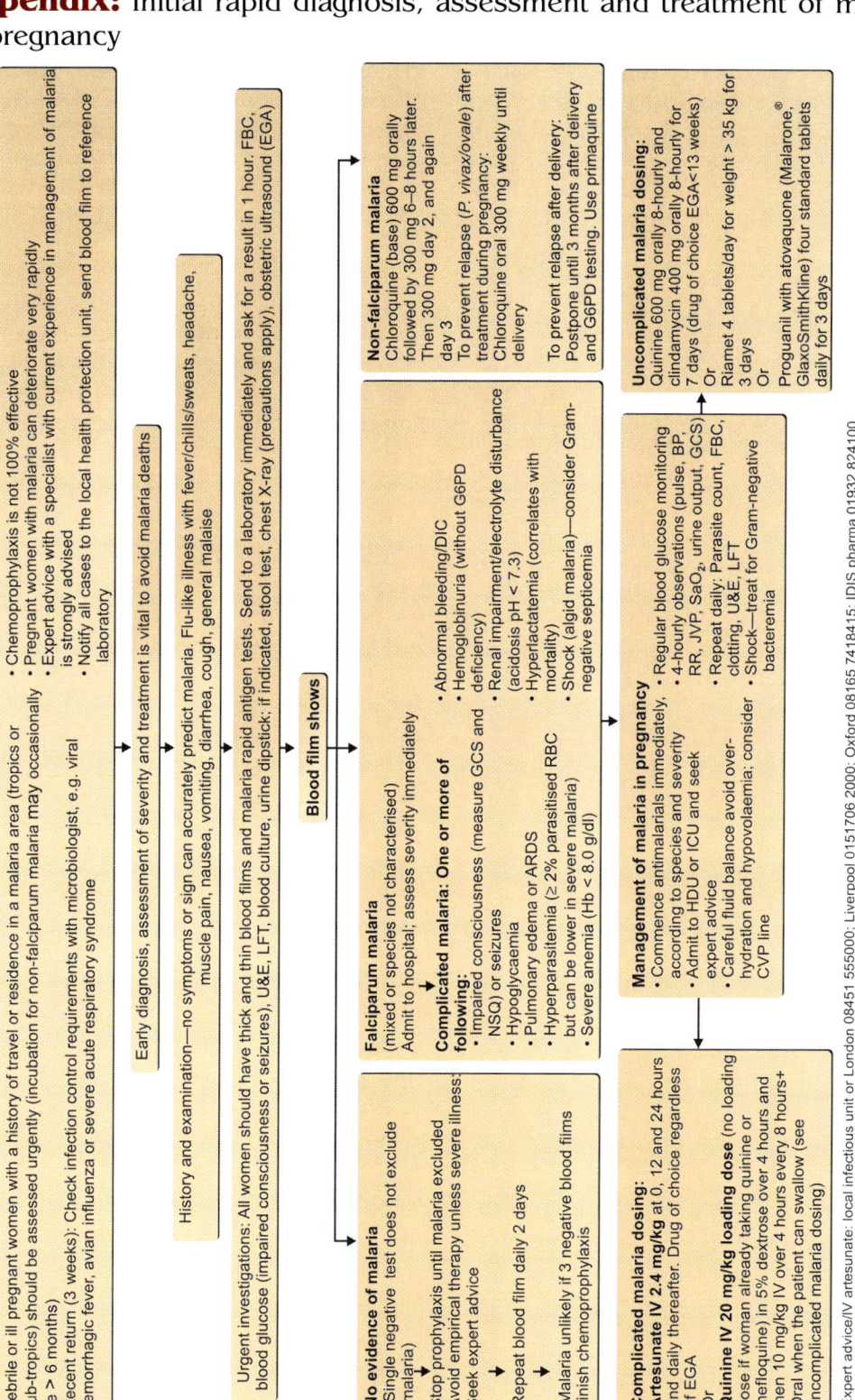

Suspect malaria

- Febrile or ill pregnant women with a history of travel or residence in a malaria area (tropics or sub-tropics) should be assessed urgently (incubation for non-falciparum malaria may occasionally be > 6 months)
- Recent return (3 weeks): Check infection control requirements with microbiologist, e.g. viral hemorrhagic fever, avian influenza or severe acute respiratory syndrome

- Chemoprophylaxis is not 100% effective
- Pregnant women with malaria can deteriorate very rapidly
- Expert advice with a specialist with current experience in management of malaria is strongly advised
- Notify all cases to the local health protection unit, send blood film to reference laboratory

Early diagnosis, assessment of severity and treatment is vital to avoid malaria deaths

History and examination—no symptoms or sign can accurately predict malaria. Flu-like illness with fever/chills/sweats, headache, muscle pain, nausea, vomiting, diarrhea, cough, general malaise

Urgent investigations: All women should have thick and thin blood films and malaria rapid antigen tests. Send to a laboratory immediately and ask for a result in 1 hour. FBC, blood glucose (impaired consciousness or seizures), U&E, LFT, blood culture, urine dipstick; if indicated, stool test, chest X-ray (precautions apply), obstetric ultrasound (EGA)

Blood film shows

Non-falciparum malaria
Chloroquine (base) 600 mg orally followed by 300 mg 6–8 hours later. Then 300 mg day 2, and again day 3
To prevent relapse (*P. vivax/ovale*), after treatment during pregnancy:
Chloroquine oral 300 mg weekly until delivery

To prevent relapse after delivery: Postpone until 3 months after delivery and G6PD testing. Use primaquine

Uncomplicated malaria dosing:
Quinine 600 mg orally 8-hourly and clindamycin 400 mg orally 8-hourly for 7 days (drug of choice EGA<13 weeks)
Or
Riamet 4 tablets/day for weight > 35 kg for 3 days
Or
Proguanil with atovaquone (Malarone®, GlaxoSmithKline) four standard tablets daily for 3 days

Falciparum malaria
(mixed or species not characterised)
Admit to hospital; assess severity immediately

Complicated malaria: One or more of following:
- Impaired consciousness (measure GCS and NSQ) or seizures
- Hypoglycaemia
- Pulmonary edema or ARDS
- Hyperparasitemia (≥ 2% parasitised RBC but can be lower in severe malaria)
- Severe anemia (Hb < 8.0 g/dl)

- Abnormal bleeding/DIC
- Hemoglobinuria (without G6PD deficiency)
- Renal impairment/electrolyte disturbance (acidosis pH < 7.3)
- Hyperlactaemia (correlates with mortality)
- Shock (algid malaria)—consider Gram-negative septicemia

Management of malaria in pregnancy
- Commence antimalarials immediately, according to species and severity
- Admit to HDU or ICU and seek expert advice
- Careful fluid balance avoid over-hydration and hypovolaemia; consider CVP line

- Regular blood glucose monitoring
- 4-hourly observations (pulse, BP, RR, JVP, SaO₂, urine output, GCS)
- Repeat daily: Parasite count, FBC, clotting, U&E, LFT
- Shock—treat for Gram-negative bacteremia

No evidence of malaria
(Single negative test does not exclude malaria)
Stop prophylaxis until malaria excluded
Avoid empirical therapy unless severe illness. Seek expert advice

Repeat blood film daily 2 days

Malaria unlikely if 3 negative blood films finish chemoprophylaxis

Complicated malaria dosing:
Artesunate IV 2.4 mg/kg at 0, 12 and 24 hours and daily thereafter. Drug of choice regardless of EGA
Or
Quinine IV 20 mg/kg loading dose (no loading dose if woman already taking quinine or mefloquine) in 5% dextrose over 4 hours and then 10 mg/kg IV over 4 hours every 8 hours+ Oral when the patient can swallow (see uncomplicated malaria dosing)

Expert advice/IV artesunate: local infectious unit or London 08451 555000; Liverpool 0151706 2000; Oxford 08165 7418415; IDIS pharma 01932 824100.
Useful information: www.hpa.org.uk/HPA/ProductsServices/InfectiousDiseases/LaboratoriesAndReferenceFacilities/1200660023262/ and www.who.int/malaria/publications/atoz/9241546948/en/index.html
Key: ARDS - acute respiratory distress syndrome, BP - blood pressure, CVP - central venous pressure, DIC - disseminated intravascular coagulation, EGA - estimated gestational age, FBC - full blood count, GCS - Glasgow Coma Score, Hb - hemoglobin, HDU - high-dependency unit, ICU - intensive care unit, JVP - jugular venous pressure, LFT - liver function test, NSQ - Neuroticism Scale Questionnaire, RBC - red blood cells, RR - respiratory rate, SaO₂ - oxygen saturation, U&E - urea and electrolytes

Index